THEMING SKILLS FOR
YOGA TEACHERS

Yoga Teaching Guides

As it grows in popularity, teaching yoga requires an increasing set of skills and understanding, in terms of both yoga practice and knowledge. This series of books guides you towards becoming an accomplished, trusted yoga teacher by refining your teaching skills and methods. The series, written by experts in the field, focuses on the key topics for yoga teachers – including sequencing, language in class, anatomy and running a successful and thriving yoga business – and presents practical information in an accessible manner and format for all levels. Each book is filled with visual aids to enhance the reading experience, and includes 'top tips' to highlight and emphasize key ideas and advice.

in the same series

Qigong in Yoga Teaching and Practice
Understanding Qi and the Use of Meridian Energy
Joo Teoh
ISBN 978 1 78775 652 6
eISBN 978 1 78775 653 3

Supporting Yoga Students with Common Injuries and Conditions
A Handbook for Teachers and Trainees
Dr. Andrew McGonigle
ISBN 978 1 78775 469 0
eISBN 978 1 78775 470 6

Developing a Yoga Home Practice
An Exploration for Yoga Teachers and Trainees
Alison Leighton with Joe Taft
ISBN 978 1 78775 704 2
eISBN 978 1 78775 705 9

of related interest

Yoga Teaching Handbook
A Practical Guide for Yoga Teachers and Trainees
Edited by Sian O'Neill
ISBN 978 1 84819 355 0
eISBN 978 0 85701 313 2

Yoga Student Handbook
Develop Your Knowledge of Yoga Principles and Practice
Edited by Sian O'Neill
ISBN 978 0 85701 386 6
eISBN 978 0 85701 388 0

THEMING SKILLS FOR YOGA TEACHERS

Tools to Inspire Creative and Connected Classes

Tanja Mickwitz

Series Editor: Sian O'Neill

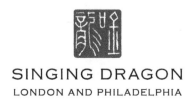

SINGING DRAGON

LONDON AND PHILADELPHIA

First published in Great Britain in 2022 by Singing Dragon,
an imprint of Jessica Kingsley Publishers
An Hachette Company

1

A CIP catalogue record for this title is available from the
British Library and the Library of Congress

ISBN 978 1 78775 687 8
eISBN 978 1 78775 688 5

Printed and bound in Great Britain by CPI Group

Jessica Kingsley Publishers' policy is to use papers that are natural, renewable and recyclable
products and made from wood grown in sustainable forests. The logging and manufacturing
processes are expected to conform to the environmental regulations of the country of origin.

Jessica Kingsley Publishers
Carmelite House
50 Victoria Embankment
London EC4Y 0DZ

www.singingdragon.com

CONTENTS

ACKNOWLEDGEMENTS

Since the very beginning of my yoga journey, I have been blessed by studying and practising with many extraordinary, wise and knowledgeable teachers, simply too many to mention here. Sreedevi Bringi and Pandit Rajmani Tigunait are two particular lineage holders whom I want to specifically honour with deep gratitude for their generosity and luminosity; I am so blessed by your teachings and wisdom. I will be forever grateful to Yogarupa Rod Stryker for introducing me to the lineage as well as the deeper aspects of practice. The appreciation and love I have for Sianna Sherman knows no bounds; thank you for your endless inspiration, wisdom and support as a guide, mentor and exemplary community leader. Thank you to the whole Rasa Yoga collective for being my yoga family, to all my fellow seekers, teachers and students alike, who are an endless source of support and inspiration to me.

Finally, this book would never have been written if it was not for Sian O'Neill, who first reached out to ask me to contribute to the *Yoga Teaching Handbook* and later suggested the writing of this very book – thank you for all your support, encouragement and patience, too!

MY STORY

I began my journey with yoga some 20 years ago. What a journey it has been and continues to be. Never could I have imagined where that very first yoga class would lead me. Though something extraordinary did happen that very first time on the mat: to my complete surprise, I found home. It wasn't that I felt at home in the practice per se. My body screamed and shook through the *asana* as I reawakened muscles I wasn't even aware existed. But the homecoming happened in *savasana* (corpse pose). It was an experience I couldn't describe in words but one of connection so deep and so familiar. Like I'd found something I hadn't even realised I'd been looking for.

Yoga quickly became part of my daily life, and after some years of dedicated practice, I was really yearning to know and understand more. I knew the practices had profoundly changed my life, but I didn't quite understand how. And this is what led me to train as a teacher. It really was more for studentship than thinking about becoming a teacher. But then I realised that I really loved sharing the practices, and for me, teaching also created the opportunity to keep learning. In my experience, the best teachers are avid students; that is certainly true of all the teachers with whom I have studied.

Now, it's interesting to think back to the first few years of my practice and the difference in my experience of how classes were taught back then and how classes are taught now. This is based on my very limited experience of classes in London. However, when I started going to classes, there was not much talk other than *asana* instruction. It tended to be *asana* straight up and down, no preamble, no closing offering other than possibly chanting *Om* at the end. This did show me how potent the practice is, as it brought me such incredible transformation simply through the *asana*. I began to change and my life as a whole started to change, as I wanted to make different choices, with practice becoming a priority. This is the immense power of the breath, the mind and the conscious movement of *prana*. But I had no awareness nor understanding of what was actually happening until I started teacher training. And even if there is much to be said for self-discovery, I have over the years really come to appreciate the opportunity to share more of what yoga has to offer in my classes in ways that are relevant to the students and their lives. I also know that if I had only offered *asana* in my teaching, I would never have lasted this long as a teacher. It is the process of finding and exploring themes that keeps it alive for me. It's rewarding for me and by extension, hopefully, for my students, too. For sure, inspiration is contagious; when we feel inspired and fresh, this will be very obvious to students, too.

In the very beginning, I would mostly focus on very basic sequencing themed around an area of the body, say the shoulders or hips. From there, my understanding of the subtle body began to grow, and for a long time I would use the *prana vayus* as the theme for practice. However, for some strange reason I had this idea that I shouldn't be explicit in explaining my underlying theme to students; rather, my theme should be felt so strongly in the practice that it became obvious. It still makes me chuckle a little when I think about this now – how I'd convinced myself that this absurd idea was something to strive for! And then I found a teacher who would always bring in beautiful readings and personal anecdotes to share in class, and I so loved her classes because I really felt she offered something more: that she was being generous with herself and her journey and that this allowed me to go so much deeper in my practice, too. And from there, I began to grow as a teacher, adding layer upon layer of the things I learned into my classes. The first time a student said to me that being in my class was like going on a journey, I felt so rewarded. This was and is exactly what I want to offer: an experience that feels like a journey where all the parts create a greater whole and a space for students to go deeper within themselves. And when we really consider all parts of the class very consciously, I believe this is what we create.

It takes time to find your voice as a teacher, and really, there is no rush. We cannot get all the things at once. It's a craft that is honed and takes time to build and grow. In the beginning, just being able to verbalise the poses takes so much practice. And so much focus. This is the essential foundation for teaching yoga *asana* classes. Really getting to know the poses, understand the biomechanics and then know how to relate this in a way that lands with the students. In teacher training, this is often when it dawns on trainees what teaching actually requires. I've often had trainees exclaim after class, 'Wow, I don't know how you do that, put so much in,' when they have just started to practise teaching. Just getting all the cues in for the *asana* takes a lot of practice. I often refer to it as painting. First, we begin with a blank canvas and some sketched outlines. As time goes on, we can add shading, then more colours and texture. It takes time and practice.

There are as many ways to teach yoga as there are yoga teachers. What I am about to share with you is just some ideas that have worked for me over the years. There is nothing rigid about the process I am about to share; rather, I hope that it will serve as a springboard for your own creative process and that you then take it forward in your own unique way. It is through expressing your own truth that you will resonate with your students and it is my sincere hope that the tools I offer will support you in doing so.

Chapter 1

WHAT IS 'THE ART OF THEMING'?

So what is a theme? A theme is anything that you choose to focus on in class. In my experience, the more you can distil and clarify this idea, the more potent it becomes. When you work it out in a precise way, it's like it becomes the essence and you can then drop this essence into all the parts of your class. As we know, something in concentrated form is stronger, right? And with theming this also brings greater clarity, both for you as a teacher and for your students.

I think of the theme as the *sankalpa* of the class. *Sankalpa* translates as resolve or intention, and the theme is your intention for the class. It holds the overall experience that you would like to share with your students. We will look more at how to find your themes in the coming chapters, but for now, let's just find an example and see how we move from an idea to a theme.

Imagine that one of the gifts you feel your practice has given you is that you are able to make better choices for yourself, and you would like to share this with your students. Now, making better choices is a great result of yoga practice; however, to make it relevant for practice, you would want to look at what it is in the practice itself that is allowing you to make better choices. So you might take some time to really think about what happens in the practice that has facilitated this change. It could be many things, but let's say you feel that the most valuable thing has been that you now listen inwards before you make decisions.

If you wanted to make this the theme for your class, 'Listen inward to have the opportunity to make better choices in the future' will be quite long-winded. Even if this is the bigger picture, you would want to make the theme quite specific and distil it into its potency. I suggest that you keep your specific theme to five words at the most, ideally fewer. Three words is great, and keeping it simple with just one key word works well, too. So for this class, you could feel into it and sense that the essence of what you want to share is 'Listen within'. Now that you have the anchor point for your whole class, this is the theme.

Where does the 'art' come in? It comes from the ability to weave the theme through the whole of the class. I'm sure most of us are familiar with what some people call the 'sandwich theme'. This is the idea that we introduce the theme at the beginning, we teach the class and at the end we mention the theme again, which easily happens. So the theme appears as two bookends or slices of bread, as it were, but isn't present through the centre or the filling.

The missing piece is the embodiment, and in my opinion, using the embodiment and the poses in very intentional ways is one of the great gifts of *asana* practice.

Bringing the theme through the whole of the class requires some refinement of skills. But what it requires most is that you as a teacher feel deeply connected to the theme. Teaching is in itself about embodiment in many ways. What you bring as a teacher is mostly non-verbal. Students learn through your presence. You know this from being a student yourself. You can really feel the teachers who have done a lot of practice and who live their practice; you know this even before they speak because they carry it in their whole being. Now, if you hold the theme strongly within you as you teach, this will also be communicated. And to do this, you need to be very clear, hence the distilled short form of your theme. So your connection comes first and foremost. I suggest that you work out your theme by speaking about it and journaling. The more thought you give it, the more embedded in you it becomes. And from this point, you start to really find the 'bhav', the feeling intention, of your class. When you have this, you can start to create with it and find the elements that help to embody and express the feeling essence of your theme.

Another important piece as you start to work and explore your theme is relevance. Why is the theme you have chosen important – what is the value of this exploration to your students? I think of a curious child asking me the question 'Why?' over and over again. So if we take our theme 'Listen within' as an example, it could look something like this:

> Listen within. Why? So that you can hear what truly resonates as being right for you. Why? When you feel aligned within, you feel more peaceful. Why? When you act from a place of harmony within, you will have a more balanced impact on your environment. Why? This contributes to a more peaceful world.

You can keep this going for as long as you wish to really go deeper with the meaning. It doesn't necessarily mean that you will offer every single idea when you're teaching; this process is really the first step and is just for you. It's a bit like a guided brainstorming where some things will really land with you and you might then offer these things as you teach. The main aim is to give you further inspiration around your theme. Then, when you come to teach, it will be so much richer. If a theme hasn't been deeply contemplated, you can find yourself just repeating the same phrase over and over again. And to be fair, this in itself is also helpful for students: repetition is a great teaching tool. But when you have given more thought to what you are teaching, you will naturally end up sharing more about it.

With exploration, you might also find that your *bhav* evolves. And from there comes the embodied exploration. How can you in your body help facilitate this feeling? Is there a pose in which you particularly feel this feeling? You can begin to craft your sequence from there. All the while, holding your theme as your intention, and whilst you do this, you will discover surges of creativity in how this can be expressed. And then you begin to add in the layers of the different parts of practice, as we will explore in the following chapters. The key is to hold the focus of your theme throughout the process; this in itself will be the gateway to new inspiration and mean that when you teach you are fully present with the theme. Then, you will discover yourself dropping into this essence through the whole class rather than just at the beginning and the end. Because it is part of you from the beginning and through the whole creative process, it will stay present with you as you teach it, too.

As with anything else in life, when we bring presence and intention to theming, it flourishes. This is what opens up portals of inspiration and creativity; this is what allows for a sense of continuous renewal.

— Chapter 2 —

THE GATEWAYS
TO THEMING

We will now look at how we can approach finding themes for classes. I have created some categories to show different approaches and entry points to theming. At times, we might find ourselves brimming with ideas of what we want to share with students, but at other times, it might be useful to look towards these different categories to ignite our inspiration and creative process. These are the main gateways that I have used over the years:

- philosophy

- mythology

- *asana*

- energy body

- natural cycles

- personal story.

Philosophy

We are blessed with such an incredibly rich tradition and many beautiful, extraordinary scriptures. Yogic philosophy is truly time-tested and holds as much relevance today as it did thousands of years ago, which in itself is remarkable and extraordinary. Much of the yoga that is portrayed in the west has sadly been reduced to only *asana* and the physical aspect of the practice. I believe we would all do great service both to the tradition and to our yoga community by offering more of the philosophical roots of yoga in our classes. The philosophy doesn't need to be lofty and esoteric at all; when the underlying principles are understood, they can be very practical, applicable and helpful to daily life. What this requires from us as teachers is that we have a genuine and also embodied understanding of the principles. We don't want to be sharing Sanskrit *sutras* with obscure translations unless we can then expand on the ideas and make them very relevant to our students. We need to have a personal relationship to what we are talking about and sharing. You have to be willing to engage with your own enquiry to really make it juicy for your students. One understanding of Tantra is that it is the weaving together of philosophy and practice. In other words, we don't want the philosophy we read and study to remain in our minds, we want to apply it in our practice and in our lives.

In her trainings Sianna Sherman, founder of Rasa Yoga, often talks about 'street language', meaning that we need to be able to translate and word our ideas in ways that can be understood not just by dedicated yoga students but by any person we might might meet off the mat, too. This is actually a great way to find out if we truly understand the meaning, as it forces us to find the very essence of what we are talking about. It also challenges us to find the relevance: how can we draw on this idea formulated so long ago and feel it help and support us in our daily life? In a sense, as the teacher you become the bridge between ancient wisdom and modern life. It is good to hold the view of the universal all the way to the very personal. You might not necessarily share your personal story in class (though you might choose to) but it is important that you have explored what your personal story with the theme is even if it is anchored in philosophy.

If you feel like you don't really 'know' much about the philosophy, just remember your time in teacher training: you most likely read Patanjali's *Yoga Sutras* and the *Bhagavad Gita*. We can return to these two texts again and again; something new will always be revealed. You might even be surprised by how inspired you feel. You could also come back to the same text but use a different translation and interpretation to find something new.

Mythology

The Vedic stories of the Gods and the Goddesses have long been a personal love of mine. That is not to say that we by any means need to limit our use of mythology to the Indian tradition; we could use any stories to illustrate a theme and a thought. You could argue that as humans we begin to understand our world through stories; from when we are young, we are told bedtime fairy tales and stories. I love this idea that, as humans, what makes us distinct is that we are a story-telling species. Stories can be very powerful in relating ideas, as, I believe, we hear stories not just with our minds but with our hearts, too. In stories, we also meet archetypal characters, and these help us to understand parts of ourselves. Some say archetypes speak directly to the soul and offer great points of reflection on who we are.

The Hindu deities all carry very distinct and particular identities that represent energies present within all of us. We can understand this even without any kind of devotional practice. The language of symbolism and archetype can be used universally to express ideas. At the same time, we always want to honour and respect the tradition in which they were born and to which they belong.

There are stories held within the names of some of the *asanas* themselves. Students might find it really interesting to understand why we are suddenly talking about 'the Lord of the fishes' or 'the eagle', for example. This is really another way into understanding the very rich tradition of yoga. The stories often illustrate philosophical or moral points. It is worth noting, however, that the same story can be told in many different ways depending on lineage and philosophical *dharsana* or school. Again, it is worth doing some research and really finding out what resonates as true for you. And what is the relevance of the story or the symbolism for your students – does it offer a valuable contemplation?

The pantheon of Vedic deities is complex and abundant. And there are many different ways to interpret it, as well as the relationships between the deities. In the more Tantric view, we can see everything beginning to take form from the two basic energies of all of the universe, Shiva and Shakti. Shiva is the all-pervading consciousness of everything, and Shakti is the power of manifestation. You could say that Shiva is stillness and Shakti is movement. They are constantly intertwined; one exists within the other. If we only had Shiva, everything would be inert, stagnant, whereas if we only had Shakti, all would be in continuous chaotic movement. In their mythological form they become the God Shiva and the Goddess Shakti, the two eternal lovers. From these two forces, the universe becomes manifest. The next layer, if you like, of manifestation is where we then find Brahma, the creator, Vishnu, who upholds the balance of the universe, and then Shiva, now in his form as the destroyer. This we can see as the cycle of beginning, middle and end that is ever-present in all of life. The three are known as the Trimurti, or the three faces of the Divine. These three Gods then have their consorts, who are three different forms of Shakti, also known as the Tridevi. They are Saraswati, Lakshmi and Durga. Then, in yet a more manifest realm, we have the Devi Loka, the realm of the Gods and the Goddesses where they now take the forms of, for example, Indra, the king of the Gods with the thunderbolt, Vayu (the wind), Surya (the sun), Chandra (the moon), etc. We can also see these manifestations as all of the elements and also all of our senses. In this perspective, it then becomes clear that all of the stories are really taking place within us. The battles and the demons are internal rather than external. With this in mind the stories become very rich soil for finding engaging themes for classes.

Asana

We can also find our themes in the embodiment and physicality of *asana* itself. The different poses carry different qualities, which in themselves hold wisdom and perspectives of understanding. As we know, the work with *asana* truly never ends. There is always more subtlety and nuance to find; it's an ever-generative process. We can start an enquiry with a single pose, or perhaps with a group of poses, and from here lead into a theme. We often approach sequencing by moving towards a peak pose, so we could choose our peak pose and then reflect on the particular lessons this pose might have for us. It might be the journey towards the peak pose that actually teaches us something. Or it might be the experience in the pose itself. There might be a particular feeling that we experience within the pose. Some poses even have themes in their names already, like 'fierce pose' or 'warrior'. It could also be that you choose to, for instance, focus on forward folds because you're teaching a class late in the evening. Then, you can come into an enquiry about the qualities of forward folds and what it is you are hoping your students find through doing them. This can then be evolved into a more specific theme.

If you were to choose a strong inversion as your peak, then you would look at a whole different set of attributes or qualities. You could focus on some of the actions you need to cultivate in both your body and your mind to practise the pose. To flesh it out into a theme, you would then contemplate how these qualities are relevant other than on the mat – how can students transform what they learn in the process into something helpful outside of their *asana* practice, too? In this way, we can not only help to bridge the gap between practice and life but hopefully help our students feel empowered, too. It is such a powerful tool to use our bodies in this intentional way – to feel how our bodies can help us shift our mind state, too, in a conscious way.

Energy body

The anatomy of the subtle body and the understanding of how *prana* moves can be a great opening for finding themes for classes. This can really help students understand how the practices work on much deeper levels than just the physical. There are several energy-body maps we can use. Some are more esoteric and others more accessible. I find working with the *panchamahabhutas*, the five great elements, an excellent way to introduce everyone to the more subtle energetic workings of the practices. The idea of the elements is immediately very tangible and easy to grasp. Most people will have a direct relationship with earth, water, fire, air and even space. As soon as you offer the elements, they'll have a sense of the qualities you mean and then you can further embody these qualities through *asana*. We even have reflections of the elements in our language: 'I feel grounded,' 'The conversation was flowing,'

'He flared up,' 'She's an airhead,' 'I feel really spacey,' etc. You can also use the elements as an entry point to the *chakra* system. Most people, whether yoga practitioners or not, will have heard of the *chakras*. They might find them a bit 'new-agey', but anchoring into the elements might ground this belief a little. The *chakras* do provide an excellent map as they really speak to all parts of our being. The *chakras* weave together our physical, emotional, mental and spiritual self. Working with the *chakras* as themes can offer a wonderful way of experiencing how our physical self can help to shift things in our feeling and mind-bodies.

Another excellent map that can provide good material for themes is the *prana vayus*. The 'vital winds' and the way *prana* moves can really help students to understand how energy shifts depending on how we choose to move. Knowing the energetic effects of *asana* is such a helpful tool, and we can then use this knowledge to help to find balance. Ultimately, we practise to become more balanced, but unless we have an understanding of how this actually works in *asana*, we won't know how. We can actually view the whole *asana* practice as a *pranayama*, as what we are doing is harnessing and shaping the vital life force. So the experience of how we move in different ways, to energise, for example, and how we choose to move to find our centre or to calm down is a very useful tool to share with students.

You could share another model, the *koshas*, in thematic teaching to give an understanding of the layers of our being and how yoga gives us an opportunity to experience and understand our wholeness.

All the subtle-body maps serve as a great way to open up discussion around the depth of both our being and the richness of the yoga tradition. We are teaching *asana* but also an understanding that we are moving much more than just our physical self in our practice.

Natural cycles

Yoga invites us to connect more deeply without as well as within. In our modern lives, certainly if we live in an urban environment, we can easily become quite cut off from nature. I often wonder whether this might be one of the reasons why we have destroyed the planet to the extent we have. Would we not be behaving quite differently if we had a more direct relationship with nature? The truth is that we are nature, there is no separation, but somehow the trajectory humanity is on seems to have separated its identity from nature. So if yoga gives us a path to wholeness, it by extension opens up this opportunity to reconnect with our environment and the natural world. Everything in nature moves in cycles and we are cyclical beings, too. We relate less immediately to these cycles in the present day as our daily activities don't have to rely on sunlight hours and what we eat doesn't have to rely on what's in season. Arguably, this contributes to issues with health and well-being. However, most people will feel nourished and replenished by time spent in nature.

Paying attention to the seasons can be a great tool for reflection. How is winter different from summer – what happens in nature and does this reflect how we feel? Do we need different things and different practices at different times of the year? Working with the seasons can be a great gateway to really reflecting on what we need to find greater balance and how our practice can help with this.

Another cycle to work with is that of the moon. I believe that coming into connection with the moon cycle is a wonderful way to connect to both nature and a sense of greater perspective. The moon can be a great way to find a connection, especially if you live in the city and don't have the opportunity to spend much time in nature. The moon's gravitational pull causes the high and low tides of the oceans. As humans we are made up from an average of 60% water, so perhaps it isn't a far-fetched idea that we might also be affected by the movements and pull of the moon. In traditions like Astanga Yoga, you are advised not to practise on the full or new moon, as it is understood that these days have a particularly strong effect on us. For women, the menstrual cycle reflects the movement of the moon, and I have heard many women say that when they have started to pay attention to the moon, their cycle has aligned with it.

Whether you or your students feel these cycles of the moon and the seasons or not, contemplating them can bring awareness to our own more personal cycles. Through everything, there is a pulsation, from beginning to end, emergence to death, expansion to contraction. This is how this ever-changing world expresses itself. So noting where we might be, whether with our jobs or within our relationships, internally or externally, can provide some support to acknowledge this ever-moving flow of the world and life itself. It also provides a beautiful opportunity to reflect on how our inner and outer worlds mirror each other and what we can do to come into greater harmony within and without.

Personal story

The final category I will use here is what I loosely term 'personal story'. I know that I always remember it when my teachers share something personal, something about their journey and their experience. It weaves into what I mentioned earlier about stories in general; we are all storytellers and we all love hearing each other's stories. This is how we relate to each other. Using our own experience is a great way to show how the teachings can be embodied and how they relate to real lived experience.

A personal story can be anything that we are willing to share that will have relevance to our students and to the practice. It can be an anecdote about how breathing more deeply helped us through a family argument or how because we are more present, we are able to catch the beauty in a small moment. It can also be about big life shifts or challenges and how our practices helped us navigate these. However, what is absolutely essential is that we only bring to class things that we have processed fully and can speak to without being pulled into the emotion of them. We don't want it to become 'the *insert your name here* show'; it must be very clear that we are sharing not to simply talk about ourselves, but rather to illustrate a point of yoga-in-action in one way or another. In the personal, we are looking for the universality – to the point within the story that students can identify with and relate to.

It can be a lovely way to connect and for students to get to know us a little better through what we share, but again, we must tread carefully so as not to become overindulgent. Students come to class for themselves, to learn more about themselves in the practice, not to hear about their teachers, so it's a fine line. It comes back to asking the question of 'Why?' again. When we question our chosen theme or anecdote in this way, it will become clear whether sharing it is of value, or not.

As has probably become clear to you by now, these aren't necessarily different categories but they interweave and can easily be connected. The idea of this differentiation is more about clarifying gateways or openings to begin to find different themes. As we then come to apply the techniques introduced in the next chapter, you will see how these different maps actually interconnect and support each other in many ways.

Chapter 3

THE THEMING LOTUS

Your Map to a Fully Integrated Class

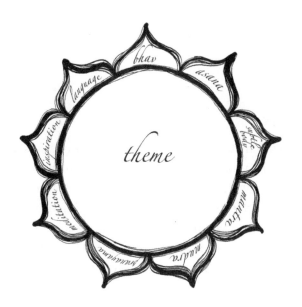

Several years ago, when I was doing work around theming, I came up with this visual and template of the theming lotus. To me, it represents a lovely way in which we can look at the unfolding of a theme into different petals or parts of a class. It gives us an overview of the different aspects of a class but also allows flexibility in terms of how much we choose to use. We can see our theme as the very centre of the lotus and then how this theme can reach out in specific ways to the different aspects of the class. To me, this theming lotus both provides an opportunity to dissect what a class can be made up of and holds within it the complete integration of the theme in every part of the practice we are teaching.

With the theme at the centre of the lotus, these are the different petals you can grow around your theme:

- *bhav*

- *asana*

- subtle body

- *mantra*

- *mudra*

- *pranayama*

- meditation

- inspiration

- language.

Returning to this metaphor of beginning a painting, first sketching and then slowly adding colour and texture, let's remember that you can add the petals gradually. Not every class needs to feature every single aspect. However, in your class planning, it might be helpful to think about what each part would be, even if you don't end up teaching it. This comes back to really working your theme, getting familiar with it and exploring it. The more you embody your theme, the deeper the connection will be when you teach.

So we come to the theming lotus once we have found a theme and distilled it into a strong one-to-five-word essence. At this point, you have done some contemplation, you might have journaled and possibly had some conversations around your theme. You feel that you have a clear message that you want to offer in your class.

Bhav

I place this at the top of the lotus as it really infuses everything else. *Bhav* or *bhavana* refers to the heart and feeling intention that we hold.

This is really what carries your theme from deep within. This is what you feel when you speak your theme out loud. This is the meaning it holds on a deeper level. This will be key to finding your way through the other petals. It might not be much different from your theme necessarily, but it might be more personal to you. For example, if your theme is 'Stand your ground', this could probably call forth a different *bhav* for different people. It could mean courage for one person; it might mean steadfastness for another. This doesn't matter; what is key is that it resonates with you and your intention in this particular instance. You could say that with the *bhav* we are looking for the embodied feeling of the theme and the message. This is what will help you find your way. It gives you the emphasis that you want to explore through all the other parts of the class.

Asana

Once you have a theme and a clear *bhav*, you can now start to investigate what pose or poses might feel most supportive in underlining your message. What are the qualities you are looking to emphasise and what would you like your students to explore? You might get a very clear sense of an apex pose that you would like to work with. It could also be a group of poses. Perhaps it's a journey you want to illustrate, a type of movement or a key action.

It is worth taking some time to explore on the mat by feeling into your body rather than just thinking about it. Perhaps you could do a spontaneous practice by simply holding your theme as your intention; you might be surprised at what evolves. This is a bit like journaling around your theme but doing it through the body instead of contemplating through writing.

This is really where you have the opportunity to build the bridge from purely teaching *asana* to adding layers of depth. We find this when we think of *asana* beyond strengthening and stretching the physical and understand how the *asanas* make us feel and cultivate deeper capacity.

Another aspect of the physical practice is that when we practise *asana*, we really meet ourselves. How we respond and react in our practice often mirrors exactly how we respond to challenges in life off the mat.

Our practice gives us an opportunity to see our patterns more clearly and the space to perhaps make different choices. On the mat we slow down, we pause, and in this pause, we have an opportunity to reflect before we react. We can watch our tendency to push, our default to opt out, our fear of slowing down, our need for distraction, whatever it might be. Feeling and knowing that we have a choice in how we respond is what gives us freedom.

And it could be that your theme directly speaks to and highlights some of these things quite clearly.

Subtle body

You could choose to either find the subtle-body connection after you have chosen your apex pose or find the energetic landscape of your theme before choosing your apex pose or series of poses. You will find the way that works best for you, and this will partly depend on how familiar you are with the energetic understanding of the practice. In the previous chapter, we looked at finding the theme through the gateway of the subtle body in which this aspect, or this petal, is already very clear.

If you aren't very familiar with the *chakras, prana vayus* or *koshas*, this could be an opportunity to learn more, as this can be very supportive in finding depth in practice and sequencing in an energetically supportive way. To begin with, you might choose to focus on the elements, as this is very relatable and accessible for your students, as well. Again, you want to take some time to explore and investigate the elements; the more you cultivate a felt sense of the qualities, the richer it will be. So when you think of your theme, does it feel like earth, water, fire, air or space? If you take it a step further into the *chakras*, where would it fit? In the first *chakra* we meet our sense of security, our physical body, our primary support. The second *chakra* holds our desires, sensuality and our feelings. Our sense of self, our confidence and courage connect to the third *chakra*. In our hearts, we find connection, compassion and love. All very different to the expressiveness of the throat, vision of the third eye and gateway to universal consciousness at the crown. In this way, the *chakras* offer such a good point of connection to finding the *asanas* that are most supportive of our theme. There are many great resources for studying which *asanas* connect to which *chakra*. We also want to remember that, ultimately, we are not looking to build the energy of the *chakras* necessarily; rather, the idea is that we want to balance the *chakras* so that they can dissolve. The idea of *laya* yoga is that we dissolve the *chakras* so that the energy, the *kundalini shakti*, can rise up freely along the *sushumna nadi* (the central channel). So when we add *chakra* awareness into our classes, we offer the enquiry into whether students might feel they have either too much or too little energy in these centres.

The model of the *prana vayus* also offers a great support in enhancing our theme. From our theme and our *bhav*, we can get a sense of how we want to shift the energy. For example, is it a practice of letting go and release (*apana vayu*), or is it an uplifting energy (*udana vayu*)? Perhaps it is about drawing in and building energy (*pran vayu*), about finding centre (*samana vayu*) or about circulating energy (*vyana vayu*). In broad strokes, you can categorise poses by where they direct energy as follows:

- *apana* – forward folds

- *pran* – backbends, laterals

- *udana* – backbends, inversions

- *samana* – twists

- *vyana* – laterals.

You can also link the *prana vayus* to the elements:

- earth – *apana*

- water – *vyana*

- fire – *samana*

- air – *pran*

- space – *udana*.

This energetic map can be a very useful entry point to sequencing your class; I have relied on it for crafting classes a lot.

Mantra

Not everyone is comfortable chanting and not everyone wants to use *mantra* in class. As with each of these petals, it is something to consider and then use if it resonates. There are many *mantras*, from the classical Vedic to the melodic kirtan-style chants. Whether you use *mantra* will also depend on your students. If you're teaching a corporate client, you will probably be less inclined to bring in chanting than if you're teaching in a dedicated yoga centre, for instance. But it might be nice to consider which *mantra* would fit nicely, even if you decide against actually teaching it in class. If you do teach a *mantra*, be mindful of how long it is. Is it manageable for students to learn? Would it be helpful to have *mantra* sheets? Maybe you just decide to sing the *mantra* yourself as a blessing for the practice. What you do want to consider offering is an explanation of the *mantra* so that your students feel that they know what they (or you) are chanting. It can be quite intimidating and possibly alienating to just hear these words in a language you don't understand, so you need to be the bridge that makes it relatable and accessible.

Mudra

Mudra means seal, and these can be made in many ways, including with the whole body, but in this instance, I will be referring to *mudras* made with the hands, known as *hasta mudra*. *Mudras* have been used within both the yogic tradition and Indian classical dance for millennia. They can be seen as symbolic but they also have strong energetic patterns. There is a variety of traditions and, just like with the *chakras*, we find different variations. In the tradition I have learnt, the five elements relate to the thumb and the fingers in this way:

- thumb – fire
- index finger – air
- middle finger – space/ether
- ring finger – earth
- little finger – water.

So through the hands, we have the currents of the elements and we can understand that how we shape and move our fingers and hands will have an effect on our subtle body. There is a whole science to how *mudras* affect the flow of energy and how we can use them therapeutically.

I also find *mudras* work very well to anchor and seal intention; this is how they can really enhance the power of our theme. If we explain the *mudra* and then return to it through the practice, it will really help to thread the theme in a potent way, even in the moments when we don't verbalise it.

Again, this might be a part of the theming lotus that really speaks to you; equally, you might not feel drawn to working with *mudras* at all. But if you already use *anjali mudra* and *jnana mudra*, do consider exploring a greater repertoire of *mudras*; you might find it a great source of inspiration and a layer that adds even more depth to your practice.

Pranayama

Arguably, breath awareness is one of the most key concepts that characterises yoga practice. To what extent we include *pranayama* practices will completely depend on who we are teaching. If we teach beginners, simple breath observation and just reminding them to breathe every so often might be the best thing to do. With slightly more experienced practitioners, we can begin to use different techniques. I would suggest looking at the subtle-body connection to find the most supportive *pranayama* practices. The breath is the most powerful tool to begin to shape, harness and direct the flow of *prana*. *Pranayama* can be added at the beginning or end. It can be used in *asana* and also as preparation for meditation.

Meditation

How and if you include meditation will again depend on the nature of the class you are teaching. Whether you will teach meditation or not, it can be helpful to think about what kind of meditation would work with your theme. Then, even if you only add a short minute of sitting, it will help you give an orientation to what contemplation to add to this short seated moment. It can be very powerful to offer some moments of seated stillness as a close to practice before the end of the class. Sitting together in stillness is a very different experience to everyone lying down in *savasana*. And at this moment, you can share a thought or some imagery that relates to your theme to anchor it once more. If you have longer and if your students are open to meditation, you have a lot of scope to explore many different practices.

Inspiration

This petal is broad and definitely open to expansion and interpretation. What I mean by 'inspiration' in this instance is inspiration from sources other than yourself; in other words, something that you have come across that has resonated with you and dropped you into a deeper understanding of the theme you are offering. This could cross over with the 'philosophy petal'; perhaps you choose to share a reading from one of the scriptures. It could also be from a book about yoga that explains something in words that resonate with you and you feel will be understood well by your students. Equally, however, you might be looking outside of the scope of yoga. Ultimately, our practice takes us into all aspects of our life, so you might choose to share something you have read outside of the yogic remit. Poetry, for example, can offer lovely contemplations for the practice. And as with mythology, poetry often reaches us at a deeper level than purely the mind; it speaks to our soul.

Language

It can be worth taking extra time to explore the language and the words you use to enhance the connection to your theme and in particular your *bhav*. What words can help you find the feeling connection? What kind of language will support the experience? For this, journaling can be helpful and also writing out key words and then finding as many synonyms as you can. In this way, your expression will become richer, and you won't as easily fall into repeating yourself over and over. This will also help you deepen your own connection with what you're conveying, and you will become even more embodied in your theme and present with the *bhav*. This is, in general, a good exercise to use to expand out of our default vocabulary and stay fresh in how we express ourselves.

So now you can see that if you look at all these aspects of a class in a conscious and intentional way, you will come up with a practice that will feel very well rounded and will offer a fully integrated experience for your students. As I have mentioned, you might choose not to use all of the petals, or they might not be appropriate in all the classes you teach. It is also important that you don't feel overwhelmed by trying to include too many things at once before you feel confident to do so. You can start small and gradually add pieces as you continue to hone your craft. These are skills to build over time – over years, in fact. But if you feel stuck in a rut with your teaching, working with this template should definitely help to revive your creative juices. And the more you think it through, the more you will feel confident and inspired by your theme. Your own inspiration is key to inspiring your students.

Over the next few chapters, we will explore how we can, through the different gateways to theming, begin to find the different petals of our theming lotus. As you read on, I encourage you to take note of your own ideas and how you might have chosen something different to what I suggest. All of it will help to stimulate your curiosity and creative thinking.

Chapter 4

STHIRA SUKHAM ASANAM

Theming Through the Gateway of Philosophy

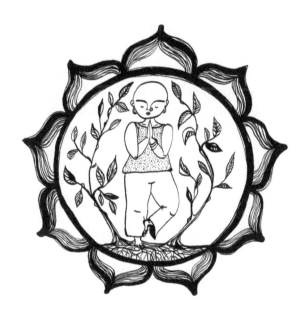

Our first theming gateway is yogic philosophy. I have chosen to begin here, as it seems foundational to everything we do. This is a vast topic and, for sure, you could ground all your classes in philosophy from here on for your whole teaching career and not ever run out of interesting themes. Some of you will have a real passion for the scriptures and diving deep. Others will have found the philosophy challenging and difficult to resonate with. Often, our relationship with a subject has much to do with the teachers we have. Yogic philosophy can be approached in a very scholarly and academic manner, but it can also be approached from a very practical point of view. The tradition is truly time-tested; the principles apply as much now as they did thousands of years ago. Much of what yoga teaches us seems universal to the human condition.

It is essential that we have a basic understanding of the different *darshanas*, or schools of thought, in the tradition, as their orientation is quite different. One big distinction is whether the system is based in dual or non-dual thought. There are the philosophies Vedanta, Advaita Vedanta and Tantra. All my primary teachers have been steeped in classical non-dual Tantra, and this is what most resonates with my experience. Hence, this is where the foundation of my teaching is based. However, as I am just offering examples, you can certainly see as we go along where perhaps, for you, other foundational principles work better. Everything can and should be adapted in ways that resonate with you personally.

For the sake of simplicity, I have decided to use one of the often-quoted verses in the *Yoga Sutras* as the theme to illustrate how we can craft a class rooted in yogic philosophy. I have chosen it for its accessibility, as almost everyone will likely be familiar with the *Yoga Sutras* from their teacher training.

Sthira sukham asanam

Sutra 2.46 in Patanjali's *Yoga Sutras* is referred to very often, perhaps because it is one of the very few *sutras* that mention *asana*. Here is the translation of the verse by Pandit Rajmani Tigunait:

A stable and comfortable posture is *asana*. (Tigunait 2017, p.223)

Unlike many of the other *sutras*, here the translations are fairly congruent and in agreement. We must remember that with Sanskrit translations and commentaries, we get huge variations and ranges of interpretations. This is due to many factors, including which era, tradition and culture the translator comes from. It is valuable to check in with a few different translations, as this also gives us an enriched understanding.

So after we have chosen our *sutra* or concept, it can be good to immediately examine our own reflections. What is it that immediately resonates for us? What questions might we have? Is there something about it that feels particularly true in our own experience? Why do we want to share it and explore it further?

Reflections

In this way, referring to this *sutra* becomes a connector between this ancient scripture and modern-day yoga practice in the west. However, it is unlikely that Patanjali was referring to *asana* as a yoga pose in the modern understanding. *Asana* means 'seat'; it can refer to both the seat we take and what we actually sit on. It can also be seen as the seat we take within our inner being. But in all interpretations, it is likely that it concerns the seat taken for meditation. Arguably, all *hatha* yoga practices work as preparation for taking our seat in meditation, so introducing this *sutra* can be a great way to introduce more of what yoga has to offer for students who perhaps only associate yoga with physical yoga practice. These ideas of taking a steady and comfortable seat can then be expanded on to begin to find these qualities in not only the whole of the practice, but in life, too.

To find steadiness within an uncertain and ever-changing world feels incredibly valuable and desirable. This is one of the great promises of yoga practice: that we can find some stability within. Of course, it doesn't matter how much we practise, things will still happen to us. We will have difficult relationships, we will lose loved ones, natural disasters will continue to happen and so on. But how we react to these outer circumstances and how we deal with them has much to do with our inner steadiness. In a similar way, finding ease within can transform our whole experience of life. If we are at peace with ourselves, the way we act and move in the world will be completely different.

Between these two qualities, there is a pulsation. Steadiness implies stillness, whereas ease carries with it a sense of flow. I like the idea of thinking of the two as the interplay between Shiva and Shakti. Shiva is the energy of all-pervading consciousness. Shakti is the power of creation and manifestation. In the mythology, Shiva and Shakti are lovers and always intertwined. And in life, everything holds these two energies. In our *asana* practice, we can find the experience of this as we move to find stillness, and when we experience stillness, we come to find that the stillness is also dynamic. Another illustration of this would be the yin-yang symbolism; each quality holds within it the other. In practice and in life, we want to cultivate the balance of both. We don't want to find so much steadiness that we become rigid. We also don't want to be so filled with ease that we lose our ground.

Bhav

So from this reflection, we can now begin to distil that our *bhav* will be to find pretty much what it says in the *sutra* itself: stability and ease. To hold the pulsation between the two.

Asana

Ultimately, we aim to find these qualities in any and every pose throughout the practice. But we can now start to think about which poses particularly lend themselves to experimenting with this pulsation. This could be an opportunity to go back to very foundational *asanas* to explore these qualities and then apply them through other shapes, too. You could begin in the very simplest way by inviting students to lie down in *savasana* and have them feel the steadiness of the ground supporting them whilst feeling the ease of the body letting go. Coming to sit, this could be the enquiry for *sukhasana* (easy pose). So in its name, this pose carries the invitation to find the '*sukham*', the good space. However, we all know that for many students, this pose is far from comfortable or easy. So now working within the pose, it can be an invitation to explore how it might be possible to find ease. Do you need to sit on some height? Or perhaps add some support under the knees or the feet? Emphasising finding '*sthira* and *sukham*' here can really open up the conversation around where we have a tendency to push through pain or put up with discomfort. How does it feel if we release expectations of how we think our bodies should be and instead truly feel for steadiness and ease within?

Tadasana (mountain pose) is another perfect opportunity to find this balance. Inherent in the name is feeling the stability of a mountain, and when we play with balancing in alignment with gravity, we find ease and a natural internal lift through our bodies.

Another way in which these qualities can be explored and experienced is by individuating them. For example, you could work with a very still and steady warrior – establishing stability to begin with and then moving into a flowing sequence to feel into the ease of movement. This could be broken down in greater simplicity, too. Have students on all fours (tabletop position) – first just connecting through the hands, stability and engagement through the arms and a long spine to explore *sthira*. Then, invite them to move freely through hip circles and to move the spine in a fluid way. After this, combine the two qualities in *marjarasana-bitilasana* (cat-cow) stretch. A similar exploration can be invited in *adho mukha svanasana* (downward-facing dog).

You could choose to teach a sequence that holds all the foundational poses as well as all the different types of poses – supine, seated, standing, balancing, inversions – to get an orientation on how to find *sthira sukham* through them all. You could also use the opportunity to work towards quite a challenging peak pose by approaching it from this perspective of steadiness and ease. For instance, if you were to sequence towards *adho mukha vrksasana* (handstand), it could be interesting to observe the point at which you feel you lose the connection, and what it is that has shifted. Is it in the body or in the mind?

Subtle body

The natural association here would be the element of earth and, by extension, the root *chakra*. You could also make it an exploration between the first *chakra* and the second *chakra*. *Muladhara* for steadiness and *svadhisthana* for flow, with an interplay between the two. In the energy map of the *prana vayus*, the stabilising force could be found through *apana* or *samana vayus*. *Apana* is perhaps somewhat more aligned with this particular theme as it carries with it the quality of release and, in this way, ease, too. With *asana* referring to the seat in physical form, in whichever way you interpret 'seat', it can relate to tending to the *annamayakosha*, or 'food body'.

As we are establishing the foundation with this first theme we are exploring, let us stay with the elements and the earth. All of the *asanas* are rooted in the earth in one way or another. In our bodies, the legs and the feet particularly relate to the earth and are the way we find stability in any pose. This goes for being upside down just as much as it does for standing poses. I often refer to our legs and feet as the 'roots'. When we activate the legs, we immediately stabilise. Again, this could be experienced within a pose like handstand, if this was appropriate for the students in the class.

Mantra

The *sutra* in itself – *sthira sukham asanam* – can be chanted as a *mantra* and is quite easy to follow, even for students not familiar with Sanskrit. As they are likely to hear these words repeated again and again, it might be really nice for them to articulate the words themselves, too. And the words carry the vibration of the qualities, as well.

Mudra

Two *mudras* immediately spring to mind to help establish this connection with the earth element. The first one is *prithvi mudra*, the seal for the earth. In this *mudra* we bring the thumb to touch the tip of the ring finger. The second is *bhumi sparsa mudra*, with the left hand resting with the palm upwards on the lap and the fingertips of the right hand touching the earth. In this *mudra*, there is also the connection between the water *chakra* in the pelvis and the root *chakra* at the base.

Pranayama

To find steadiness and ease, the breath is absolutely key; this is where it all begins. It can be very useful to introduce the concepts of steadiness and ease to beginners when it comes to them exploring the breath. In the beginning, we first just need to remember to breathe, as we often hold the breath when we concentrate without even realising it. The following step is to establish an even breath. Taking time to establish a simplified *sama vrtti* variation of breath with an equal inhale and exhale can be a wonderful way to feel into the qualities of *sthira* and *sukham*. The full form of *sama vrtti* would include equal counts of inhale retention and exhale retention as well, but this is a more advanced practice. For beginners, it is useful to do the simplified form of *sama vrtti* practice whilst lying down; for those who are more experienced, you can offer it in a seated position. And then through the practice, the remembrance of this continues to be a point of reference. Are we still holding the steadiness and ease in the breath? Re-establish it and breathe it into the whole of the body in whichever *asana* you are in.

Meditation

This theme serves as a perfect vehicle to introduce meditation in a class. Ultimately, these are the qualities we need to be able to sit for meditation. We can feel the pulsation of moving into stillness, how finding the ease in the body through movement helps us find the stability to be still. It can be as simple as sitting for one minute and just being with the outer body steady (*kaya sthiram*) whilst feeling into the *sukham* (good space) within.

Inspiration

In this case, we already have our clear inspiration from the *Yoga Sutras*. It could be a nice continuation on the source of this theme to offer more from the *Yoga Sutras*. What happens when we find steadiness and ease in our pose? In *sutra* 2.48 Patanjali offers:

> From that
>
> perfection of a yoga posture,
>
> duality,
>
> such as reacting to praise and criticism,
>
> ceases
>
> to be a disturbance.

This translation and interpretation is by Mukunda Stiles (Stiles 2002, pp.28–29).

So this is a very rich area to explore. How would it feel to not be pulled off centre by all the polarities and dualities in our lives – to experience equanimity in this way?

Language

Here, we can take some of the key words – steadiness, ease, earth, flow – and begin to find the verbs and more words that call forth these attributes.

Bringing it all together

So now we have all the petals of our theming lotus, we can begin to thread them together. At the beginning of the class, we can open by introducing the *Yoga Sutras* of Patanjali in a few words and then share this chosen verse with some reflection on why this is of value for us all, off the mat as well as on it. Now, with some sense of the meaning of the words, the *mantra* can be introduced, and this will help to charge the atmosphere for the class. During the *mantra*, one of the *mudras* can be offered; perhaps *prithvi mudra* at this stage, so it becomes familiar. After the chanting, students can be invited to lie down, to feel the steadiness of the earth and to simultaneously invite ease into their bodies through letting go. From here, breath awareness can be gradually introduced, followed by guidance into *sama vrtti* breathing. Then, start to come into the sequence with continued awareness of the breath, the ground beneath and the ease within. As a reminder of the steady earth, *prithvi mudra* can be added to poses where the arms are free and extended, such as *anjaneyasana* (low lunge) and *virabhadra* (warrior pose).

Tadasana can serve as a place to return to between the more dynamic and moving sequences to again find *sthira*. *Vrksasana* (tree pose) is a great pose for exploring both the steadiness and the ease, as you need both to stay balanced. As you move through backbends, you can really hold the steady connection in the legs as you encourage the ease in the heart space. Then, it can be very interesting to explore how the dance between *sthira* and *sukham* moves very differently in seated forward folds; it is worth pointing out, as a reflection, that different bodies will find connection to these qualities in very different ways and in different poses.

At the end of the *asana*, students can be guided into a seated meditation for as long as seems appropriate for the particular class. They can return to *prithvi mudra* as the focus becomes a steady body (*kaya sthiram*) and the good space within. Once everyone returns to *savasana*, they can be invited to witness how they feel now in comparison to how they felt at the beginning of the class. To finish, you can return to the *mantra* and hold the *bhumi sparsa mudra* as a reminder to stay steady as you move from the class back into the world. This is also an opportunity to offer some words of encouragement, contemplations or affirmations on how the benefits of the practice can be taken into daily life.

OVER TO YOU!

- Which scripture has made the most impact on you and why?

- What relevance does yoga philosophy have to your daily life?

- Which are the top three yogic principles you feel would make the biggest difference in your students' lives?

- Take each of these principles and explain them in street language; find examples of how they work in modern life.

- Now, from what you have written, create three succinct (one to five words) themes – and then begin to play with the theming lotus. You can choose just three 'petals' for each theme.

Chapter 5

THE GODDESS SARASWATI

Theming Through the Gateway of Mythology

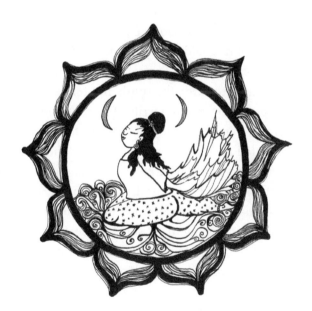

In the Vedic tradition, the deity for learning and wisdom is the Goddess Saraswati, so she seems to be a good example to use here.

The story (in one of its many different renditions and allowing for some poetic licence) goes that, before creation, Brahma, the creator, was sat with the whole of the universe in front of him; he had all of the ingredients for the cosmos but it was all a big soupy mess and he didn't know what to do with it. He needed help and he realised that the only one who could help him was the Great Mother, the Great Goddess, the *Maha Devi* herself. So he started to make offerings of *mantras* and prayers to the *Maha Devi*, asking for help. Eventually, he started to feel a deep vibration from within; he opened up his mouth and out of his mouth manifested Saraswati herself. She had a bright radiance all around her and her whole being was vibrating to the sound of *Om*. She was riding a pure, white swan, and in her arms, she held a *veena* (an Indian instrument similar to a lute) and *mala* beads. Her beauty was otherworldly, ethereal, divinity embodied. Saraswati took one look at the messy soup of creation and, with one magical sweep of her hand, she organised all the three worlds and the whole of the universe. Brahma was completely taken aback by her eloquence and her wisdom, as well as her beauty. He was quite besotted. Once Saraswati had finished her work, she walked off towards the east to practise her *mantras* with the sunrise. Brahma was too curious; he realised she probably wanted to be on her own, but he couldn't help himself and grew a second head to follow and watch her. When Saraswati realised this, she changed direction; she walked towards the south and tended to her creative spark by sitting down to draw and write. Again, Brahma couldn't help himself; he sprouted another head to be able to follow her. Saraswati, a little more irritated now, got up and walked with her *veena* towards the waters in the west and started to play some *ragas*. And Brahma once again grew a new head to follow the sweet music. Saraswati was at this point pretty annoyed; she rushed off towards the north and buried her head in the *Vedas*, hoping to get some peace. Shiva had for some time been following the events from afar; he became more and more upset with his friend's unsavoury behaviour. So when Brahma popped a fifth head, Shiva had finally had enough and he intervened, cutting off Brahma's fifth head and telling him he had to stop disrespecting the *Devi* in this way.

Some time later, and with much apology, Brahma did manage to convince Saraswati to marry him. At first, he was ever so happy, as he was completely besotted with his new wife. However, after some time, Brahma came to realise that married life with Saraswati wasn't quite what he had hoped for. His wife was often completely preoccupied with her constant learning and creating. He would wait for her at breakfast, and she would always be late because she took so long with her morning *mantra* practices. When she eventually appeared, she would sit down with her nose buried in one of the scriptures rather than pay Brahma attention. She was notoriously late for all their social engagements because she would get so lost in her music or her writing. She forgot to come to dinner because she was busy finishing her painting before the sun set. Then, one day, there was a big ceremony, a *puja*, to which all the Gods and the Goddesses were invited. Brahma and Saraswati were to play an integral part in this ceremony. Brahma told his wife that she must not once again embarrass him in front of everybody by being late. Saraswati reassured her husband that she would be there on time and told him not to worry. But, lo and behold, as it got to the time of the start of the *puja*, Saraswati was nowhere to be seen. Brahma was beyond furious and he had had it once and for all; rather than wait once again, he denounced his wife and, being the creator, he created himself a new wife in the form of Gayatri. When Saraswati eventually arrived to witness this, she cursed Brahma to never be worshipped by anyone, since he had disrespected her in this way. And even to this day, there are in fact only two temples in the whole of India – and you can imagine how many thousands of temples there are all over India – that are dedicated to Brahma.

So in this story, we can see some of the empowerments of Saraswati. She is the Goddess of all wisdom, learning, creativity and the arts. The name breaks down into *saras*, which translates as water, lake, and *vat*, which means to possess, to have. Together, they translate as 'the flowing one' or 'she who flows'. So Saraswati is what we experience as the flow of inspiration. Those moments when we are completely caught up in what we are doing or creating, inspiration carries us and it is almost as if something greater flows through us. This is Saraswati Shakti. She is also what holds all communication; Sally Kempton talks of the internet being a Saraswati invention (Kempton 2013). You could say that she is both our inner wisdom and our intuition. If you experience writer's block, Saraswati's energy is what you want to call in or awaken within you.

Bhav

The underlying feeling is finding a sense of flow and awakening inspiration, whether this is to learn or to create. There is also an understanding that creative flow is inherent in our being and to find it requires deep listening and presence.

Subtle body

Thinking of the *panchamahabhutas*, there is a natural affinity between Saraswati and water. In the *chakra* system, this bring us into *svadhisthana*, the second *chakra* in the pelvis. However, there are other *chakras*, too, which align well with Saraswati. The throat *chakra* for vibration, sound and creative expression, which are all Saraswati empowerments; as well as *ajna* and *sahasrara chakras* for wisdom and insight. You might choose one, two or at most perhaps three *chakras* to focus on in one class. Another avenue in the map of the *prana vayus* would be *vyana vayu*, which embodies this sense of flow, water and the multiple locations we found with the *chakras*.

Asana

So for this particular class, let us make the main focus the second *chakra*, and this can now inform the choice of *asanas*. With the *bhav* of finding flow and the *svadhisthana chakra* orientation, it seems natural to focus on the pelvis and hip-opening. This is also where many find tension and holding, physically and energetically, so it can be a great way to explore finding flow where you might experience tightness or restriction. *Eka pada rajakapotasana* (pigeon) could be a good apex pose to have in mind; with the water element as guidance, this could playfully be advanced into *naginyasana* (mermaid), for a more intermediate class. The hip joint lends itself to finding flow, as it has such an extensive range of movement to explore. Let's say we choose to sequence towards *naginyasana*. This pose requires a lot of preparation to externally rotate the hip and stretch the front of the thigh and hip flexor, as well as mobilise the shoulders. On the whole, there could be an emphasis on joint movement and joint mobility as joint health is reliant on fluidity.

Mantra

Saraswati brings the world into being through the sound of *Om*, so this is a natural *mantra* to bring in for the practice. The *bija* or seed *mantra* for Saraswati is *Aim*. So the two syllables could be chanted together: *Om Aim*. If it feels appropriate, the whole root *mantra* could be offered – *Om Aim Saraswatyai Namaha* – and chanted a number of times.

Mudra

The 'wisdom seal' or *jnana mudra* would work nicely, as Saraswati is the Goddess of Wisdom. This *mudra* is familiar to many, so adding it to the poses within the *asana* sequence would be fairly straightforward. Another *mudra* to play with for flow is *ap mudra* for the water element, where you bring the thumb to the tip of the little finger.

Pranayama

Circular breathing could be a nice exploration of the focus on flow and release of stagnation. In circular breathing, we aim to soften any roughness in the breath as well as to flow from inhale to exhale and exhale to inhale seamlessly. So we cultivate a smooth and uninterrupted flow of breath.

Meditation

As a meditation, you could offer anything from simple breath awareness, following the flow of breath, to something intricate and creative with Saraswati as the inspiration. Let me offer you one example that ties in the theme to try and see how it feels.

PRACTICE

Please find a comfortable and steady seat, where you can feel your spine lift with ease and without effort. Take a few deeper breaths and let your breath be the bridge that carries your awareness from the external world to your interior. Feel your outer body settle into stillness. Bring your awareness to the flow of your breath. You are not shaping or changing the breath; you simply come to observe the natural movement of your breath. Stay aware of the movement of your breath whilst you connect to the base of the spine, the root *chakra* space. Then, move your awareness to the crown of the head and the seventh *chakra* space. As you feel the flow of your breath, now start to trace the movement of the exhale down the spine from the crown of the head to the root. Then, follow the inhalation from the root up to the crown. Stay at ease, stay effortless, as you trace the flow of breath along your spine and the central channel, *sushumna nadi*. In mythology, the Saraswati River is seen to symbolise this central energy channel in our being. As we free up the flow, we free ourselves up to our innate creativity, insight and wisdom, all the qualities of Saraswati that we find within us. Continue and let yourself bathe in the flow of Saraswati's blessings. You are simply surrendering to the flow; allow yourself to receive. After a while, you might find that the flow of energy releases itself from the pattern of the breath; let it take you, trust the flow.

When you are ready to come out of meditation, breathe a little deeper, let your chin drop lightly towards your chest. Inwardly offer gratitude for any deeper insight or understanding that might rise out of the meditation, honour the sacred space you have been in and slowly blink your eyes open and return to your surroundings. With Saraswati's blessings of creativity, this would be a great time for some free-flow writing to bring yourself out of meditation if you are able to do so. To complete the practice, you can chant either the Saraswati *bija mantra* or the root *mantra* whilst holding *jnana mudra*.

Inspiration

When using mythology, the symbolism or the stories provide a great information resource with much to share. You might also be able to find some texts or poetry dedicated to the deity you are focusing on that you could share in the class.

Bringing it all together

Almost everyone loves a story, so if you feel comfortable sharing a story, it is a great way to begin a class. You can make it longer or shorter depending on the time available. But if storytelling feels too ambitious, another way to use mythology is to simply share the empowerments of the deity. It is also important to make it accessible and really emphasise that the archetype of the deity can be used as inspiration to cultivate and invoke these qualities within. It doesn't have to have any devotional aspect (unless this feels natural and comfortable).

With the scene set by Saraswati's story and/or empowerments, the practice can then begin with the chosen *mudra* and *mantra*. From there, start to come into an easy flow of breath and movement. To begin to connect with the pelvis and the hips, the practice could also start in *supta baddha konasana* (reclined bound angle pose or cobbler pose), where everyone can feel the breath all the way into the second *chakra* space of the pelvis whilst also becoming aware of the hip joints. Students can be invited to explore where they might be experiencing physical stickiness and how breath with movement can help them to release into flow through warm-up circular movements of the joints. Flowing between *asanas* through the sequence can be invited, even a free flow to let inner creativity lead the way. You could introduce a *virabhadrasana* flow (warrior flow) with *virabhadra 2* (warrior 2) as the starting point, first with the arms sweeping and flowing, then moving between *viparita virabhadrasana* (reverse warrior) and *parsvakonasana* (side angle pose) and perhaps taking it into *trikonasana* (triangle pose) with the top arm moving in circles or into *ardha chandrasana* (half moon pose). After creating a simple sequence of flow, it can be nice to invite students to continue to their own breath and rhythm for a few moments.

A *virabhadrasana* sequence (warrior sequence) would also be a good way to warm up if you choose to go with *naginyasana* as the peak pose.

The practice can be completed beautifully with meditation and a return to the *mantra*. To conclude, come back to a reminder of the empowerments of Saraswati and how to continue remembering and paying attention to these through the rest of the day or week.

OVER TO YOU!

- Which story or deity are you most familiar with?

- Did you have a favourite fable or fairy tale when you were little? What about it did you particularly love?

- Find an archetype that resonates with you right now. This could be one of the Vedic deities or you can choose something like the Magician, the Warrior, the Healer, the Hero/ Heroine, etc. – let yourself be playful!

- Contemplate how channelling this archetype might be helpful. Think of a scenario where you have felt this archetype move through you, or perhaps a scenario where you wished you had felt more of this archetype.

- Create a theme based on this archetype and choose which three or four petals of the theming lotus would support you to integrate the theme.

Chapter 6

WARRIOR NOT WORRIER

Theming Through the Gateway of the Subtle Body

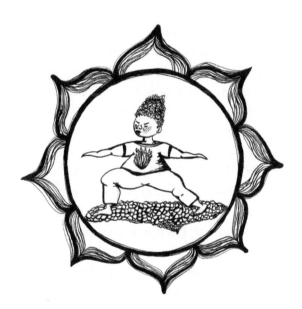

Yoga practice invites us to experience a greater sensitivity towards our subtle layers of being. In the western world, there isn't much invitation to acknowledge or honour our energy body, whereas in the Eastern traditions, this is a widely accepted and understood premise. An awareness of the subtle body can be introduced through the physical body and, as previously stated, by working with the five elements, which feel accessible to most of us.

To choose a theme related to the subtle body, let us think of something that will be useful and of help to our students in an immediate way. Many people come to yoga practice because they hope to find greater harmony and balance. Often, the motivation is to find a way to de-stress. You could argue that much of our culture is very heady – we identify with our minds more than with our bodies. There is an emphasis on resolving issues with rational thought and logic, but not so much on listening to our gut feelings. As we have already explored the earth element and the water *chakra*, let us now move towards the navel centre and *manipura chakra* for our next theme and weave in some of these thoughts.

Manipura translates as 'lustrous gem' or 'the city of gems'. This is where we connect to our sense of self, our energy, our strength and our courage. Fire also has a stabilising quality, and the navel is often referred to as the centre. The quality of fire can help us draw from our busy, scattered and stressed-out minds into our centre. Here, we can find our inner resilience and steadiness. So let's use the play on words of 'Warrior not worrier' as our theme, as this will be immediately relatable and most likely an appreciated metaphor.

Fire in itself has this ability to transform. In Ayurveda, the strength of the digestive fire is a key concept in finding overall health. You could argue that on a subtle-body level, this is equally true. We need a healthy fire to both digest and assimilate our experiences, just as we do our food. Just like our digestive fire helps us transform the food we digest into energy, our energetic fire helps us digest our experiences and transform them into wisdom. A healthy balance in *manipura chakra* also builds confidence in ourselves. Exploring this can illustrate really well how through an embodied practice we affect all parts of our being – mental as well as emotional. When we feel worried and stressed, it is unlikely that we will be able to shift our state by thinking our way through it. This is where coming into our breath and our body becomes so helpful. And the more familiar we become with being able to make this shift, the more empowered we become in our lives by finding our way back to centre when we are challenged or pushed. When our inner fire burns brightly, we are able to digest our challenges and rise up to meet them, grounded in our centre.

Bhav

From the theme of 'Warrior not worrier', the most prominent feelings that arise are ones of steadiness, strength and resilience. The image of a warrior conjures up someone who is strong in themselves, ready to leap into action and meet challenges head on. The image of the warrior really carries a very strong *bhav* in itself. This would be a good direct anchoring point to use during the class to remember all the qualities you want to invoke. There is the archetypal quality of the warrior that speaks on a much deeper level than just words, and this will carry through for all the students, too.

Asana

By natural extension of this theme, you will want to include the warrior poses in this class. If you are teaching a beginner's class, the *virabhadrasana* sequence could well be a peak sequence to work towards by breaking down alignment points and actions. This could work really well, as it is informative in how alignment anchors stability and biomechanics generate strength on a physical level. Working with the core lines of the body will also tie into *manipura chakra* awareness.

In a more intermediate or advanced class, deeper activation of *manipura chakra* can be introduced. *Bakasana* (crane or crow pose) and *parsva bakasana* (side crane) are great activators for the third *chakra* and also require the mental attitude of a warrior: courage, confidence and willingness to take up the challenge. These are also poses that can offer breakthrough moments, the moments when you finally 'get' the pose and it feels like an achievement. Of course, getting into a particular yoga pose really is just play and not the 'yoga' in itself. However, the experience of overcoming fear, for example, can be a great confidence boost. And framed in the right way, this experience can be brought off the mat into life as well. *Asana* is by no means the only way that this can be achieved, but it is one way.

Mantra

The *bija* or seed *mantra* for *manipura chakra* is *Ram*. Ram is also famously a warrior and incarnation of Vishnu in the epic *Ramayana*, so this *mantra* can be introduced with both in mind. The *chakra bija mantras* are better chanted quickly in repetition (*Ram-Ram-Ram-Ram-Ram*, etc.), as this is when you get to feel the resonance of the consonant at the beginning; it is the 'R' that resonates at the navel. This also feels quite activating, which is very suitable in this instance.

Mudra

Agni mudra is a powerful *mudra* for cultivating the fire element and connecting to *manipura chakra*. To take *agni mudra*, you bring your left hand in front of the navel with the palm facing upwards, draw the four fingers of your right hand into the palm and, with the thumb pointing straight upwards, place the side of the right hand into the left palm. This *mudra* is also known as the *shiva lingam mudra*, as it resembles the *shiva lingam* worshipped in Hindu temples as the formless form of Shiva. In this way, it also ties in nicely with using the *virabhadra* poses as Virabhadra the warrior is one of Shiva's manifestations. Holding this *mudra* with the *mantra* is very powerful and strongly activating for the warrior spirit within.

Pranayama

Kapalabhati, or skull-shining breath, is a practice that brings a very clear awareness to the third *chakra*. It's a great *pranayama* to introduce, as it can be broken down for beginners, and the intensity of the practice can be built to suit the level of the group. As an introductory practice, it is nice to simply sit with one hand just below the navel and start to practise pumping the exhale out. With more experienced practitioners, the number of rounds can be increased and then inhale breath retentions can be introduced after each round.

Meditation

It is very powerful to meditate with an awareness at the navel centre. If the class only allows for a short time for meditation, you might choose to simply sit for a few minutes resting the awareness at *manipura chakra* and observing the sensations here. For a more extended practice, either *nadi shodana*, alternate-nostril breathing, or a *kriya* called *prana shuddhi* can be a wonderful gateway to enter the practice. Both practices focus the attention at the third eye. In *prana shuddhi*, you follow the breathing in the same pattern as in alternate-nostril breathing, but you simply do it as a mental exercise. As you trace the breath in this way with your awareness, the practice is very subtle yet deep. Once you have awakened the energy at the third-eye centre and harnessed the *prana* here, you can guide it down to the space behind the navel. You can invite imagery around the colour yellow for the third *chakra* or visualise a flame. Always remember that not all students are visual; some will feel and sense rather than see.

PRACTICE

Please find a comfortable seat where you can remain steady and lift your spine tall. Let your hands rest with the palms facing down on your thighs to ground the energy and allow your elbows to relax. With the outer body steady and relaxed, begin to feel the flow of your breath. Notice how the breath is moving through each nostril like two separate lines of breath. Notice also how the inhale begins a few inches below the nostrils. The inhale then rises up through the nostrils and to the third-eye point, the midbrain, where the left and the right streams meet each other. With this awareness, we will now begin to move the breath as we would in alternate-nostril breathing. Start by feeling the exhale move out through both nostrils to a few inches below the nose, inhale through both to the third eye and then, on the following exhale, trace the breath out through only the left side. Inhale through the left to the midbrain, exhale out through the right side, inhale through the right nostril and exhale through the left. Continue in this pattern. You can imagine it like a pyramid shape moving the breath to the peak and then down the other side.

As you continue with the practice, you will notice an awareness building at the third-eye point, which will gradually become stronger. You might feel it as a strong energy, sense it as a vibration or see it as a growing light.

Once this third-eye awareness has been established and feels potent, release the focus of the breath and simply stay with the energy here at the third eye. After a few minutes, you will start to move this light, in whichever way you experience it, down towards the throat, towards the heart and finally to rest right at the back of the navel. Let this journey take however long it needs; you might experience it as a quick transition or a slow journey. Once it is resting at the navel centre, feel this energy take the shape of a bright and steady flame. Feel how this flame holds your centre, your strength, your power and your courage. This is the flame of energy, empowerment and vitality in the whole of your being. Resting your awareness here in this flame reminds you of all the moments in your life when you have felt fully yourself, grounded and strong. As you stay with this, you also rest in knowing that all these qualities are inherent in you and always available.

When it's time to come out of the practice, feel your body breathing and take a few deeper breaths. Keep your eyes closed as you bring your palms together and rub your hands vigorously together to create some heat between the hands. Once the hands feel quite hot, bring your hands over the navel and feel the awareness here and then cup your hands over your eye sockets, breathe here and slowly blink your eyes open.

Inspiration

In our modern lives, there are so many readily available examples of everyday warriors. So many living inspirations of people who have stepped forward into their lives courageously despite many challenges and hurdles along the way. And often, we get the most inspiration from real-life heroes who show us by example that we can step up in our lives, too.

What also comes to mind for me with this theme is the adage, 'Worrying is like praying for what you don't want.' Often, worry creates an incapacity to act, it holds us back from doing, it can even feel paralysing. This is where the *Bhagavad Gita* can support us with a reminder that was as applicable centuries ago as it is now. Inaction is also action; in other words, not taking action will also cause *karma* or have a consequence. This is true within you as much as it is true in the world. We know of the impact that stress has on our nervous system and how this impacts our whole being in every way. So if we can find our resilience and our centre, this action will have a huge impact on our interior. And how we feel within ourselves informs how we conduct ourselves in the world at large. We all know that if we feel stressed, we are more likely to snap at our family members or colleagues. If we are overcome with worry, we are less inclined to be fully present for our loved ones when they need us. When we're off-centre, we are more likely to make less constructive decisions on the whole. Connecting to *manipura chakra* helps us to find our centre and also our sense of self. In this way, we build trust in ourselves that we are able to meet the challenges that come our way; we start to feel secure, knowing that we have the inner resources we need to get through.

Language

Look at motivational language: how can we motivate to spring into action like a warrior? Also, think about a sense of directness in how you speak; this holds the energy of fire. To speak like fire will feel very different to the fluid language of water. Write a list of all the qualities you feel a warrior has and this will give you lots of words that could enrich how you instruct the poses.

Bringing it all together

At the start of the class, you introduce the theme and explain how embodiment can be a great way to not only get out of the head, but also change the mind state. You then guide students to begin to find a connection to their centre. As we know, warriors will move from their centre, not from their head. To help with this, you could introduce *kapalabhati* right at the beginning of the class. This will also quickly shift the energy and bring everybody to the present for the practice. Once students feel this connection to the power of the navel centre, chanting a few rounds of *Ram* might feel more accessible.

You could choose to do some core activation in the *asana* right at the beginning. For beginners, it can be good to do some variations lying down, like the 'yogic bicycle' for example, where you lie on your back, lift the knees over the hips and upper body, and then alternate opposite elbow to knee whilst the other leg stretches out. Another way to feel into the core connection is *navasana* (boat pose), with which you can get into many creative variations, such as crossing the ankles and pulsing in and away from the thighs, toes touching the mat and then reaching up to the sky or twisting elbow to opposite knee, to name a few. Once you get into downward-facing dogs and *vinyasa*, you can add some *eka pada* (one-legged plank) variations like drawing the knee towards the chest, perhaps even with a longer hold to really get the heat and determination to build. As you build your sequence, whether you are working towards a warrior sequence or some *bakasana* variations for the more intermediate students, you want to keep reminding them of their connection to their centre and their inner warrior qualities throughout. Also, doing the yoga in itself requires a steady focus; this illustrates in a wonderful way how we can let our worries drop away whilst we are staying fully present in the practice.

At the end, you can offer students a reminder of how strong and resilient they are; hopefully they can now feel themselves as embodied warriors ready to face any challenges they might meet as they leave the class.

OVER TO YOU!

- Which map of the subtle body most speaks to you and why?

- Considering that many people in modern society suffer with sleep disturbances, how could you call on subtle-body understanding to support better sleep? How could you create a general class with a universal theme that also helps to address this?

- For each of the five elements think of a verb (e.g. earth – to ground):

  - earth

  - water

  - fire

  - air

  - space.

- From each of the five verbs, craft a class theme – stay succinct and get creative!

Chapter 7

OPEN YOUR HEART

Theming Through the Gateway of Asana

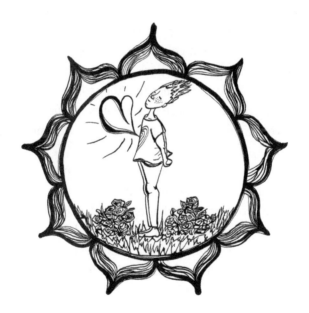

The way we teach yoga in the west is most often *asana* focused, so we tend to approach our classes from that perspective. In teacher trainings, students are offered different ways to sequence their classes depending on what style or lineage the training is rooted in. There are styles of yoga where the sequences are set, such as Astanga or Sivananda. Then, there are other trainings that offer a more universal premise. The orientation for sequencing can vary. You could have an aim to offer a class that includes all different postures and adheres to a certain flow from beginning to end, or you could sequence with an apex pose in mind.

In this instance, we will work with the idea of a peak pose, as this can help us build a more specific theme, which is the particular emphasis of this book.

So to continue to explore different effects and a different direction, let us this time choose a backbend as a peak pose. We will go with *urdhva dhanurasana* (full wheel or upward-facing bow) as our peak pose and, as always, hold the understanding that this can be modified as needed depending on the students in the class.

So what might be experienced in *urdhva dhanurasana*? It feels expansive; it opens the front body, the chest and the heart space. It can feel exhilarating and energising. And what is needed to be able to do the pose? We have the particular physical demands of the pose: the shoulders need to be open, spine lengthened, thighs stretched, legs strong, to name a few. What could some of the challenges be? Tight shoulders, weak wrists and lower back pain are some examples, as well as fear: this pose can be unfamiliar territory for many. At the core of being able to move into this pose is the ability to open your heart. So let's make this our theme, to create a class that offers something beyond just *asana* focus.

What does it mean to open your heart? Why might your heart not feel open? Here are some thoughts and enquiry that these questions take me into. We live in a culture that very much values rational thought and logic. We deem things to be true if we can find empirical knowledge and science to support it. On the whole, I think you can generalise that feelings are considered inferior to intellect, or at least less reliable. There is also a lot of emphasis on intelligence in terms of the mind and valuing this, but there is not much support offered in terms of our emotional intelligence. On the whole, we are valued in society as productive beings but less so as feeling beings. When we find ourselves in deep emotional states, there is a lot of conditioning that tells us to 'Get over it,' 'Move on,' 'Get on with it,' etc. So perhaps it's no wonder that our hearts close down a little...or a lot.

I feel that yoga practice can be an opportunity to become coura-geous enough to feel more. In my experience, practice offers us the glimpses of our eternal unchanging self and this becomes our steady anchor. We dare open our hearts more, because we know on a deeply experiential level that we are not our feelings. We don't have to be as afraid that the feelings will swallow us whole, because we know our true essence will stay the same and hold it all. Emotion can be seen as e-motion or energy-in-motion. Some would say that what is problematic is when the energy gets stuck, as it doesn't get expressed; it doesn't get to move through. If we can keep our hearts open and let the emotions move through us and feel deeply, we will become more connected within and without: to source, to ourselves and to each other.

Bhav

What is the feeling of an open heart? This might be very different for each individual, and perhaps this could actually be the enquiry you invite – to simply feel your heart space. What is alive in your heart right now?

Subtle body

Here, we have the obvious connection to the heart *chakra: anahata chakra. Anahata* means 'unstruck', and I find this so beautiful – that regardless of what happens to us, our heart remains whole and untouched. Sometimes the heart is referred to as 'the place beyond all sorrow'. Though this, of course, implies that we have layers to our heart experience, that there is the heart that feels everything and then the heart that holds it all, that remains untouched. Perhaps this is where the understanding of heart and spirit intersect. This also mirrors the understanding of love and unconditional love. There is the love that exists in relationship to someone or something, but then there is the understanding of love as the very core of our being. Please just sit with these ideas and see how they land for you. There are many different understandings, and ultimately, we all have to be guided by our own experience.

Mantra

We can perhaps generalise that most of us feel connection to love in some form through our hearts. The simple *mantra Aham Prema* holds the understanding that 'I am universal love,' 'I am Divine Love.' This is a beautiful and simple *mantra* that is easy to share in class.

Mudra

The heart *chakra* relates to the element of air. For a simple and familiar *mudra*, you could offer *jnana mudra* (the wisdom seal), as the index finger relates to the element of air. You can also see this symbolically as the individual heart connecting to the universal source energy (symbolised by the fire element in the thumb). For a more intricate *mudra*, *hrdaya mudra* is lovely. *Hrdaya* also means heart. Here, with the palms open, you move the tip of the index finger to the base of the thumb and then take the tips of the middle and ring fingers to the tip of the thumb. Rest the backs of the hands on the thighs. If the students find this *mudra* comfortable, you can return to this *mudra* in the *asana* practice as well.

Pranayama

In general, a focus on the inhalation has both an energising effect and a connection to the heart. In the *prana vayu* model, *pran vayu* relates to the heart. The inhale has an expansive quality; in other words, the quality of opening up space. *Viloma* practice can focus on interrupting either the inhale or the exhale. But here, we will focus on the inhale. *Viloma* means to 'go against the natural flow' and it is a great way to build breath capacity. This is a practice that can easily be introduced to beginners as an extension of breath awareness if practised lying down.

PRACTICE

Please lie down on your back with the knees bent and feet to the floor, hip-distance apart. You can begin this practice with some simple breath awareness. Lay your hands low down on the abdomen, just above the pubic bone with the two hands separate – not touching each other. Breathe into where you feel your hands; feel the lower abdomen expand with the inhalation. You might also feel a broadening of the lower back into the floor. Imagine you are filling your pelvic bowl with breath. Take five to ten breaths here. Then, move your hands to the side ribs so your palms are on the lower ribs on the sides of the body and the fingers point in towards the centre. Breathe into where you feel your hands, and you can even apply a gentle pressure with the palms as resistance to activate the breath a little more here. Feel how the ribs expand away from each other on the inhalation and draw back on the exhalation. Really centre the breath in the middle of the torso in all directions: to the front, to the back, to the sides. Again, take five to ten breaths here. Finally, move your hands up so your fingertips lightly rest just below the collarbones. Make sure your hands and arms stay relaxed; you just want the hands here as a reminder that you are now directing the breath to the top of the chest and the top of the upper back. Once again, breathe here for five to ten breaths. Once you have completed the cycles of breath, allow your arms to rest with the palms up by the sides of the body.

You will now come into the *viloma* practice, where you will divide the inhalation into three parts. You begin inhaling into the abdomen, just one third of the breath, and then pause for a short moment. Continue to breathe the second third of the breath into the middle of the body and then pause again. Finally, breathe all the way to the top of the chest and the full capacity of breath; pause here. When you exhale, breathe out slowly and smoothly all the way to empty. Take a regular inhale and exhale before you repeat the practice again. You can move through five to ten rounds of this practice. Make sure that the pauses feel completely comfortable so that you stay at ease the whole time. There should be no sense of tension or panic whatsoever during the breath retentions. When you become more familiar with the practice, you can omit the regular breaths in between and simply continue through from one round to the next.

Meditation

In the *Chandogya Upanishad* there is a beautiful passage which reads:

> The Self, who can be realized by the pure in heart, who is life, light, truth, space, who gives rise to all works, all desires, all odors, all tastes, who is beyond words, who is joy abiding – this is the Self dwelling in my heart.
>
> Smaller than a grain of rice, smaller than a grain of barley, smaller than a mustard seed, smaller than a grain of millet, smaller even than the kernel of a grain of millet is the Self. This is the Self dwelling in my heart, greater than the earth, greater than the sky, greater than all the worlds. (Easwaran 1987, pp.126–127)

This provides a beautiful inspiration for meditation at the heart centre.

PRACTICE

Find a comfortable seat, whether on a bolster or a chair, or if you prefer, lie down. Be sure to be comfortable and at ease. Feel where your body meets the ground and rest into the support of the earth. Sense the vastness and spaciousness of the sky above you. Now, bring your awareness to your heart, the connecting point between heaven and earth. Here at the very centre of your chest, sense, feel or see a bright seed of light. This light is the brightest light in all of the universe. As your awareness rests here, start to feel this light gradually become stronger and start to expand. The light begins to fill the whole of your chest. Slowly, it radiates outwards beyond the chest and starts to fill the whole of your body. As the light grows, it becomes so strong that it even shines out beyond your body and into the world around you. Rest here, bathing in the light of your own heart for as long as you are able to – as long as you wish.

When it is time to come back, feel this light gather back into the centre of your heart, back into its seed. Hold the knowing that this light is ever-present. Gently bow and honour the light of your heart before you come back into your breath and body. Breathe a little deeper, and when you feel ready, softly blink your eyes open and return to the space where you are.

Inspiration

The wisdom of the heart has so much to offer us. One interesting contemplation in terms of what we identify with is to consider where we gesture towards when we indicate 'I'. I would generally assume that you will bring your hand over your heart space when you either introduce yourself or express how you feel. So even if we think we identify with our rational minds externally, I would argue that this is not where we intuitively feel that our real self resides.

The heart *chakra* is also seen as the great connector. It is where we connect the most material and tangible parts of our being with the more subtle realms. In the *chakra* system, the heart is the centre between the lower and the higher *chakras*. It is also the heart that connects our inner world with the outer world. We see this very clearly through the element of air, as our breath weaves between the exterior and interior in a very direct way – linking inner and outer.

So opening our hearts means us opening up to connection in all ways. Opening our hearts also means opening up to the qualities of love, kindness, compassion and acceptance inherent within the heart. These are all qualities that enhance both our own lives and the lives of others. And aren't they, too, qualities that are so desperately needed in our world right now?

Bringing it all together

The entry point of *asana* can offer a great opportunity here to bridge the gap between the understanding of yoga as only a physical practice and how it is so much more. It is a chance to explain how we physically benefit from backbends as a way of creating more space for the breath and releasing shoulder tension, for example. However, reflection on how this actually feels can be quite profound. Working with the heart centre is powerful. Some students might be resistant to language such as 'open your heart', but you can offer this in many ways. It can be to open your heart so that you breathe more fully and feel better. And as you move through the practice, more reflections on what an open heart means can be offered. There is also the more tangible and practical reference of the breath as the connector of the inner and outer world.

This is a theme that you could quite skilfully weave from outer to inner connection through the class. You might choose to start by talking about backbends and their physical benefit: how many of us, due to life-style, experience tightness in the shoulders and don't breathe as fully as we can, due to posture. The three-part breathing practice is a great way to get connected to the breath, for both beginners and more practised students. Then, moving into shoulder release through warm up and into the *asana*, you can offer more about the energy map of the body and the heart qualities that we also open to in backbends. The invitation to feel how the heart space feels 'right now' can be sprinkled through the whole practice as you progress towards your chosen peak pose. With more experienced students, you might have *urdhva dhanurasana* and variations thereof as your apex, but if you are teaching an evening class or a generally gentler class, the peak might be a supported *supta baddha konasana*. Let's remember that 'advanced' practice is about depth of presence, not physical accomplishment; this is especially appropriate to remember whilst connecting to the heart. In fact, lying in supported stillness might for many feel far more challenging and unfamiliar than 'doing' an active pose.

If you offer the invitation to feel through the practice in this way, it will pave the way for students to be receptive to dropping into the heart-centred meditation by the end of the class and perhaps chanting the *mantra*, too, even if this wouldn't be part of their regular practice. It can be quite extraordinary how *asana* practice opens us up and expands understanding from an experiential level.

OVER TO YOU!

- What is your absolute favourite *asana*? How does it make you feel? How can this feeling translate into a *bhav* and a theme?

- Choose three peak poses – one backbend, one twist, one forward fold.

- For each of the poses you chose, write a short paragraph about their power and breakthrough potential – the essence of what they hold.

- Create a succinct theme for each pose; begin to create a class with each student using at least two of the theming lotus petals.

Chapter 8

CARRIED BY THE BREATH

Theming Through the Gateway of Personal Story

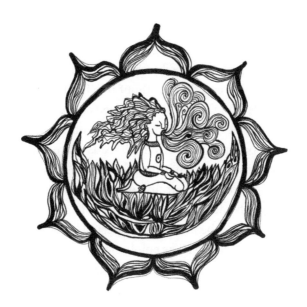

One of my teachers once said that you teach more by who you are than by what you say. What he was getting at was that most of our communication is non-verbal and that we really carry the depth of our practice with us. I have certainly felt this: with some teachers, you feel their presence before they even begin to speak, perhaps even as soon as they enter the room. And often, it is also about personal resonance. I seek out teachers who, I feel, in their teaching and being, speak directly to who I am. That does not mean that they have to be like me at all but that there is something about them which resonates with me. I can relate to them and I feel they can relate to me, too. And when I hear more about their personal story, this sense of having a relationship increases.

Using a personal story to frame a theme works well for many reasons. First, it can really help to bridge the gap between practice and life; it can help to illustrate how yoga is actually about how we live our lives rather than being isolated to doing some shapes on a sticky mat. Second, we all love a good story or anecdote. I think that lived experience sinks in on a deeper level than something that is just an idea or a concept. In fact, the story helps us contextualise and embody the principles. It might well be different for you, but I remember the personal anecdotes the most – they often stay with me for a very long time. They also help with relatability. As teachers, we are humans having a human experience as much as our students are.

There are, however, some things to be mindful of when sharing a personal story in class. You need to be sure that you have processed the content – that you can share without reliving the emotion so that you can be very clear in your delivery. It needs to be not about you but about the message you want to get across or the understanding that this lived experience brought you to. Which leads on to the 'Why?' Why are you sharing the story? What is the relevance? And what is the more universal idea or lesson that your unique story holds?

Going through the dissolution of my marriage and separating from my husband was one of the most intense periods of my life. It required a lot on a practical level as well as emotionally and energetically. I was initiating change that my heart knew was the only way forward but that was challenged by everything and almost everyone around me, including my young children who were impacted the most. From this time, I have the most vivid and visceral memory, which is the feeling of my whole body being on fire. All I could do to get through it was to breathe deeply through my whole body so I could hold the fire and not be consumed by it. This is what got me through – my breath. And this is when I realised the true impact of my many years of practice. I truly feel that there is no way I would have managed that period of my life if

I hadn't been so practised at breathing well. I would have numbed out or run away; I would not have been able to stay present.

So I can speak from my heart and share about the very real impact of being able to breathe through challenge and heartache. Now, if I were to choose this as my theme for a class, I might not share in great detail or share as much as I have shared here. I can talk about it in a more covert way, yet be very real as I share my story, and through my truth, connect with my students.

Bhav

The feeling, in essence, is of staying present by breathing deeply, regardless of the challenges you are facing: to feel the fire and keep breathing through it.

Subtle body

When we experience intensity, it is easy to freeze – to feel paralysed and immobilised. It can often mean holding our breath, too. When we breathe deeply, we help the circulation of energy. In this instance, I feel that the breath creates a circulation where the intensity could close the system down. This idea could connect to *vyana vayu* in the subtle body. We can also consider the idea of expanding into space; can we find the spaciousness around a sense of density where we meet obstacles?

Asana

As I lean into the feeling essence of the story and the teaching it carries, the embodiment of that would hold both the spaciousness of the breath and the element of fire. In other words, the embodied experience of withstanding the fire and still finding the space to breathe. There are, as always, many paths you could take with this. My imagination takes me to feeling an intense, demanding pose and staying present with the breath within it. This could be something like a challenging arm balance, perhaps *bakasana* or *astavakrasana* (eight crooks pose) for a more advanced class. For beginner or intermediate students, you could find a similar quality in a deep twist like *parivrtta utkatasana* (revolved chair), for example. To follow the story, you would want to frame the practice with deep connection to the breath, which we can do through the chosen *pranayama*.

Mantra

When life brings us intensity and fire, we can either fight against it or we can surrender into acceptance. This does not in any way imply passivity but rather an active acceptance of what is, which allows us to meet it head on rather than trying to reject reality. I sometimes feel this, as an offering up to what is. Offering myself up to the reality that is so that I can then show up fully. This theme of being able to stay with the fire and intensity makes me think of the fire ceremonies where every offering into the fire is followed by the *mantra swaha*. It carries with it this understanding of offering our experience up to something greater than we are, to the universe, to Source, to the Divine – however you personally frame it.

This *mantra* could be introduced through chanting at the beginning of the practice and then returned to as an internal *mantra* to be reminded of, especially when attempting the more fiery *asanas*.

Mudra

This practice brings focus to holding space for ourselves within all we meet in life. To hold the spaciousness within the intensity, you could use *akasha mudra*, the *mudra* for the element of space or ether. You take this *mudra* by bringing the tip of the middle finger to the tip of the thumb. It is a *mudra* that can easily be threaded through the *asana* practice whenever the hands and arms are free.

Pranayama

Connecting to the breath is always key at any point in the practice, but this theme will have even more emphasis on this. You could start with the simple practice of either lying in *savasana* or being supported by props if they're available, and coming into breath connection. You could use this time to first observe the breath, paying attention to where it moves in the body and where it moves less, before then starting to deepen and shape the breath. Invite an enquiry: do you tend to hold the breath? Is the breath more shallow in the chest or deep in the belly? What is the rhythm of breath – fast or slow, even or disrupted?

Throughout the whole practice, breathing the *mantra swaha* can serve as a continuous reminder to breathe deeply into all that is present.

Meditation

In meditation, this theme can be an invitation to sit with discomfort. It really serves as a reminder that this path is not always about just moving towards the 'love and light' experience but is also about truly embracing the icky, challenging, tough, uncomfortable parts of ourselves. Can we hold space for that, too, without running away?

PRACTICE

Please find a comfortable and steady seat. Take a moment to settle the body. You can gently move from one sit bone to the other and sway a little backwards and forwards to find your centre. Roll the shoulders up towards the ears and down and back to relax around the shoulders and open up the top of the chest. Take a big breath in and exhale through the mouth. Begin to scan your body from the top of the head, slowly moving downwards. As you move through the body, notice any places you discover that have tension or holding. Allow the softening with an internal offering of *swaha*. If you meet places of tenderness or aches, again return to the *mantra* as a way of acceptance – 'I hold space for this,' *swaha*. Once you have scanned all the way down to your feet, bring your awareness to the breath at the nostrils. Feel the sensation of breath just on the inside of the nostrils. Then, begin to move your awareness up to the bridge of the nose with the inhale and down again with the exhale. After some rounds like this, begin to follow the inhales all the way up to the third-eye space and the exhales back out again. Once you establish a greater awareness in the third eye, stay and rest there and let go of tracing the breath. Now, allow yourself to sit with what is and what arises. As thoughts, feelings or sensations arise, allow them to release with the *mantra swaha* – offer it up. Continue for a few minutes or longer.

When you are ready to come back, take a deeper breath, exhale and release your chin towards the chest. Bring the palms to touch and honour your experience. Then, begin to blink your eyes open softly and reorient yourself to your space.

Inspiration

In the *Yoga Sutras*, the fifth *niyama*, the final internal observance, is *Isvara Pranidhana*. This has been translated in many ways, but the essence of surrendering holds as a through line. *Isvara* translates as Supreme Being, Unchanging Reality, True Self or God depending on the interpretation. And *pranidhana* has many meanings, including fixing, applying, meditation and prayer. So there is this sense of offering oneself up to a greater truth or reality. Perhaps a sense of resting oneself into something more all-encompassing; this can be so helpful, especially when the immediate reality feels testing and challenging. It is also helpful to feel this sense of a greater perspective when we are really caught 'in it' with our experience, and I truly feel that breathing deeply helps me do that. And the breath itself carries a teaching of being held by something greater than our own unique individual self. Because we are not in charge of how many breaths we take in our lifetime, each breath we take is truly a gift given to us. As a very devotional practitioner myself I love the idea and imagery that each of our inhales is the exhale of the Divine and our out-breath is the in-breath of the Divine. So the Divine is breathing us all the time.

Language

This theme will carry with it a continuous return to remembering to breathe, to stay present and to keep showing up. It will require gentle encouragement to tap into inner reserves of resilience and reminders to trust in your own capacity. It is also an opportunity to remind students that even though we each have our own struggles and challenges, we can find support from each other, breathe together and hold space for each other in this way.

Bringing it all together

The invitation of this class is to breathe into our courage to stay present with the intense challenges we might face in life. It is an invitation to practise this skill to prepare us for those times in our lives when we are put to the test. We begin in the simplest way, by practising this skill of breathing fully and deeply without any other distraction as we lie down. We can also offer a personal intention: to practise this for a particular area or situation in our life. This could be a relationship challenge, a situation at work, an inner conflict, whatever it might be; you can offer your students the chance to inwardly set this personal intention. And as you guide them through the practice, the offering will be to hold space for all that is experienced and, often, a return to the *mantra: swaha*.

The practice can be a slow steady build from the breath awareness in supine at the start and become more and more engaged as the fire builds. Perhaps you begin by bringing awareness into all parts of the body, finding movement from the feet, all the way up. You can offer simple joint rotations as you move through and invite this sense of radical presence into every part of the physical presence. From here, you can build into more or less fiery salutations depending on the group you are teaching, before progressing into poses that call for deep breath and fully committed presence. This presence can then be continued into the release of the more demanding poses in the cool-down part of the sequence. The remembrance is to stay fully present with all of it and ride the waves of sensation, just as we want to stay awake to the continuously fluctuating circumstances in our lives.

At the end of the class, the effort and energy of the practice can be offered as a honouring of the personal intentions set at the beginning. Again, this really helps to bridge the practice and life off the mat, and to hold the reminder that, ultimately, we practise to live more fully and to become more skilled at living in a more fulfilled way. This can at times require us to make very difficult choices and meet a lot of resistance, but, ultimately, it is for our soul evolution. This is why we strengthen ourselves through the practices and tools of yoga. And when we can stay present through challenges, discomfort and that which is painful, it allows us to experience joy, happiness and love more fully, too.

OVER TO YOU!

- Think of a situation where your yoga practice has been of help and support to you and write about how you experienced this. Remember, it does not have to be dramatic or deep. It is important that it is something that you have processed and are no longer triggered by. Finding support for everyday occurrences, such as dealing with people on a crowded bus, can be really helpful!

- Can you draw out a universal experience from your own personal one? How would this translate into a class theme?

- Now, from this theme, play with creating a full theming lotus and stay curious as to how it can evolve into all aspects of the class.

Chapter 9

FULL MOON PRACTICE

Theming Through the Gateway of Natural Cycles

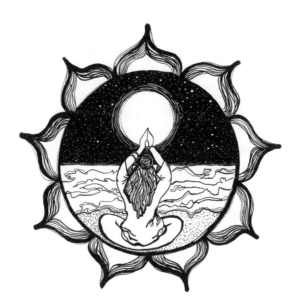

As we know, yoga means to yoke, to bring together, to connect. This practice feels more important than ever in a world where we are so disconnected in many ways. Our modern lifestyle means that we can, in many ways, create the conditions we want rather than needing to fall in line with the rhythm of nature. Since the invention of electricity, we have been free from a reliance on daylight, for example. Our days can be as long as we wish them to be. We are less seasonally challenged, as we can easily moderate the temperature to suit our needs, whether it is freezing cold or boiling hot outside. We can get pretty much any vegetable or fruit regardless of time of year, as food can be flown across the globe from the country in which it does happen to be in season.

Of course, we have begun to realise that all this convenience does have huge costs in many ways, especially for the planet. On so many levels, the dominant culture has been one of extraction and oppression, with a complete disregard for reciprocal relationship or karmic understanding of giving and receiving.

Ultimately, this does not serve anyone, as this way of living comes at the expense of the true connection, which you could argue is the only thing that makes humans truly thrive.

Becoming more embodied through our practice serves as a way to become more connected. As we start to practise, we become more aware of the connection between our mind and our breath, our breath and our body, our body and our mind. As we get a sense of the interconnectedness of our inner system, this also opens us up to the interconnectedness of all things, globally and universally.

Something that seems to have happened through our evolution is more and more separation – as though humans aren't nature but are apart from it. We live as though we can somehow be independent from nature rather than reliant on it. A juxtaposition of seeing humanity as civilised and nature as unruly, wild and not as valued or valuable has been created. I feel quite strongly that this disconnection is the root of many of our problems. This idea that we can tame nature and extract from it without giving anything back is ultimately not serving us. On many levels, it is causing us suffering.

With this in mind, I truly believe that coming back into relationship with nature is deeply healing. After all, we are nature, not separate from it. However, this isn't always easy or obvious, particularly if we live in urban landscapes. One access point to feeling into the rhythm of nature, wherever we might be, is to come into relationship with the moon and her cycle. And with the moon there is such an immediate reflection on our inner cycles, too – this energy of waxing and waning. In relationship to the moon, we can start to feel into how our energy might move: when we feel more external and lit up like the full moon and when we feel more internal like the hidden dark moon.

And, of course, the moon is always full; it's just that all of her isn't always visible to us. Just like we are always whole, although sometimes part of our wholeness is hidden in the shadows. And this experience of wholeness is what the yoga practices can help us discover, or uncover, I should say.

Bhav

The feeling this theme invites is wholeness, the sense of the full moon illuminating all parts of our being. The invitation is to rest into the knowing that all that we need is already within us.

Subtle body

With this invitation to wholeness, my mind immediately takes me to the *prana vayus*, specifically *vyana vayu*. *Vyana* is the circulatory movement of *prana*; it moves energy into all parts of our being. So metaphorically, it lights up all parts of our being, just as the sun lights up the whole of the moon during the full-moon phase.

Another take on it could be to introduce the idea of the *koshas* and how our wholeness is made up of these five different bodies, or sheaths, which are in a continuous dance with each other. The *kosha* model is a beautiful way to understand the depth of our being and the depth of our lived experience.

Asana

To connect with *vyana vayu*, a focus on laterals and inversions works well. There is a sense that we want to move into expansive poses where we can really enliven the energy through every single cell and part of our body. Through embodiment, we want to practise embracing all parts of who we are. This will be the parts of us that move with ease as well as the parts of us that might feel tender, tight or stiff.

Vasisthasana (Sage Vasistha's pose or side plank) or *visvamitrasana* (Sage Visvamitra's pose) variations could create good apex poses that can be modified in ways that are suitable for the class and students. *Visvamitrasana* carries the embedded wisdom of being the 'friend of the universe' and this idea of befriending all parts of ourselves to become whole. For a beginner's class, great peak poses could be *trikonasana*, as it radiates out in all directions with a sense of fullness, or *ardha chandrasana* for a slightly bigger challenge. Naturally, *ardha chandrasana* ties in with the moon theme in a lovely way.

Mantra

One of the *Shanti mantras*, the *purnamadah mantra*, beautifully connects to this experience of fullness. It is a longer *mantra*, but it can easily be guided through call and response.

Om
Purnamadah purnamidam
Purnaat purna-mudacyate
Purnasya purna-maadaaya purnamevaa-vashisyate
Om Shanti Shanti Shanti

That is whole.
This is also whole.
From wholeness emerges wholeness.
Taking wholeness from wholeness,
wholeness indeed remains.
Peace, peace, peace.

It really speaks to how we are never not whole; we perhaps just fail to see it. This *mantra* is an exquisite offering for coming back into remembrance.

Mudra

Hakini mudra is a beautiful seal that invites a balancing of the five elements as well as a sense of spaciousness. We press the four finger and thumb tips of each hand against each other to create a sphere-like shape. Symbolically and energetically, we are connecting all parts of ourselves. What I love, too, is that this shape that the hands are making is quite like the full moon. When we use it within the *asana* practice, we can imagine holding and moving the moon in this way; it can get really creative.

Pranayama

We can see the cycle of the breath as mirroring the cycle of the moon. We have the inhale, which builds and expands like the waxing moon, and the exhale, which releases and softens like the waning moon. This idea equates the top of the inhale with the full moon and the end of the exhale with the dark moon. With this idea, gentle inhale retentions can be built into the *asana* practice at appropriate moments.

Carrying through this idea of illumination and insight, I would offer an alternate-nostril practice with inhale retention.

PRACTICE

Find a comfortable and steady seat, where you feel your seat grounded and a sense of ease through the rest of your body. Allow your spine to lift with lightness and ease. Take a few moments to settle and bring your awareness to the flow of your breath. Prepare for alternate-nostril breathing by taking your right hand and resting the tips of your index and middle fingers at the third-eye centre, with your thumb ready to block the right nostril and your ring finger prepared to block the left nostril. In the third-eye space just behind where your first two fingers are resting, imagine the luminous full moon shining. The pattern of the breath will be 1–1–2–0, which means inhale and inhale retention for a ratio of one, exhale for double that length and no exhale retention. You can start by guiding the following counts:

Inhale – count of three or four

Inhale hold – count three or four

Exhale – count six or eight

Exhale retention – zero

Begin the practice by exhaling through both nostrils, inhale again through both and then exhale through the left to the chosen count of six or eight. Inhale through the left nostril for three or four, follow the stream of breath up to the visualisation of the full moon at the third eye and hold the breath for the given count in this space. Exhale for double the count through the opposite nostril. Inhale through the right, and continue the practice in this rhythm. Continue for as long as you wish until you feel a clear connection to the energy at the third eye. You can finish the *pranayama* by exhaling through the left nostril and then sitting for a while, basking in this third-eye moonlight. The *pranayama* could also be preparation for the following meditation.

Meditation

The full moon is energetically a very potent time for meditation. For some people, the full moon can feel intense, and many report sleeping difficulties during the full-moon nights; meditation can be very soothing. This meditation can be practised independently or with the *pranayama* as preparation, in which case you can move straight to the second step of this practice.

PRACTICE

1. Begin by settling your body into a comfortable seat. Become aware of the flow of breath through the nostrils. Feel how the inhale begins a few inches below the nostrils and moves up. Initially, follow the breath from this point up to the bridge of the nose and back out. Once you have established this connection, lengthen the pathway up to the third eye and feel the right and left streams of breath meet here at the top of the inhale before the flow moves back out with the exhalation. Continue until you feel the third eye energetically light up.

2. Now, move the illumination from the third-eye space towards the back of the crown of the head, the point also known as the

bindu. See this light as the full moon shining over the lake of your mind. Notice the waters of the lake of your mind and allow them to gently become more calm and still.

3. As you sit, you might experience thoughts, like ripples over the water. Allow them to fall away and be absorbed back into the still lake. Feel yourself resting back into the soothing and nourishing moonlight.

4. To return, gently move your awareness back to the breath, let the chin drop towards the chest and, when you are ready, blink your eyes open and reorient yourself to the space you are in.

Inspiration

The moon represents our intuitive and feeling self in many traditions and also in western astrology. In our culture, there is, in general, less emphasis and value given to nourishing these qualities. Coming into relationship with the moon herself can help us nurture this relationship within and move towards experiencing ourselves as more whole. There is also a beautiful shadow play with the moon: as she moves through the cycles, more can be revealed and then concealed, which so beautifully illustrates how we are, too. What is being called forth to be revealed out of the shadow? What parts of our wholeness are being concealed?

Language

With this theme, I would allow for lots of space between instructions to allow students to fully embrace and listen to their own experience. There is an abundance of metaphor that can be tapped into with the moon and the moonlight: 'Radiate the moonlight through your body', 'Feel the illumination of the full moon in the whole of the pose', 'Invite the light to shine even into the darkest corner', and so much more – you can really let your imagination run with the imagery.

Bringing it all together

This class is an invitation to look up and watch the moon; if it is cloudy, it is an opportunity to feel the moon behind the clouds, knowing she is still shining brightly. Often, students will have been feeling the effects of the moon but perhaps not realised it. Asking students if they have noticed the moon, been feeling a bit crazy (as in the word lunatic, which is derived from the Latin word for moon, *luna*), not been sleeping well and so on is also a lovely way to connect with everyone at the start of class.

The *mantra* and the *mudra* offer a beautiful invocation for the start of the class, which can be dropped back into throughout the *asana* practice. The word *purna* can become an anchor – inviting the wholeness and fullness of experience. *Hakini mudra* can be added to many of the *asanas*, with an invitation to imagine holding the full moon within it. For example, you can try playing with *hakini mudra* in *virabhadra 1* (warrior 1): on an inhale, raise the arms, hold *hakini mudra* up towards the sky and straighten the front leg, and then bend the knee and bring *hakini mudra* in front of the heart. You could play with circling your arms while holding *hakini mudra* as you move in and out of *asvatasana* (horse stance pose or Goddess pose, with the feet wide, toes turned out and knees bending over the ankles as the hips lower with the spine upright). As you move towards the floor in your sequence, you can add a *salabhasana* (locust) variation with the arms extended forwards and the fingers meeting in *hakini mudra*. And *hakini mudra* can be added in seated poses by holding it in front of the heart or extending it overhead before forward folding.

You can offer the idea of the 'peak' of the flow being like the energy of the full moon and how the rhythm of the cycle is inherent in how we practise. The warm up is like the waxing phase of the moon, and then we move towards the fullness of the most vigorous *asana* and then wane again, with the cool down and *savasana* being like the dark, peaceful sky of the new moon.

The meditation offers a lovely way to soothe the mind and subtle body, especially if we are feeling the intensity of the full moon. To complete the practice, a return to the *mantra* will feel really nice, as the meaning of it has now become a more fully embodied experience. At the end of the class, you might suggest that students look for the full moon as they leave the practice space. This gives a nice way to integrate the practice into the rest of the day or the evening. And, further, the theme gives an invitation to continue to reflect on the cyclical nature of being and the rhythms of nature we are a part of.

OVER TO YOU!

- What do you notice about yourself in relationship to the natural cycles? Are you affected by the seasons or by the moon?

- As you read this, what season are you in? What are the characteristics of this season? What do we need, in general, to feel more balanced during this season?

- Now, begin to elaborate your reflections into a full class or even workshop using the theming lotus.

Chapter 10

GOING FORWARD...

Now that we have taken a journey through several different class-theming gateways, I hope you are finding that ideas and inspiration are brewing. Many times, we spontaneously feel what it is that we want to share in our teaching and in our classes; the themes naturally arise. But for those times when we don't feel inspired, it is great to have some back-up inspiration to draw on. It is a good idea to keep a journal to work your themes and jot down ideas in. I highly recommend that you keep a list of possible themes that you can add to whenever good ideas arise. Then, on those days when you feel void of inspiration, you can look at the list and you will be sure to feel at least one of your ideas jump out at you and grab your imagination. Inspiration isn't a constant; it comes in waves and often works in mysterious ways, so we want to capture it when we can. Often, just a small spark of insight can birth a whole new pathway and trajectory. And when in doubt, the tradition itself always offers support through the texts and scriptures.

Building on a theme – drop-in classes

In drop-in classes, it can be nice to create a series of classes that build on a theme. This can help to build community and encourage students to commit to coming back, as they will be on a continued journey with you. You can use any of the gateways to build your series. If you would like to introduce yoga philosophy to the class, an exploration of the *yamas* and the *niyamas* tends to be a popular themed series. This can be a great opportunity to really bridge the gap between this ancient wisdom and modern life. You can find ways to guide how these principles are relevant, even in the way that we practise *asana*. For example, what does *ahimsa* mean in how we breathe, how we choose to move, how we allow the inner dialogue to run us – and then, how do we translate that into how we move and act in the world?

If you are teaching a beginner's class, it could be helpful to have different groups of *asanas* as your starting point for a series of classes. This way, you could really break down the alignment points and biomechanics to give students a good grasp and foundational understanding of the poses and how to move both into them and within them. And then, with your theming skills, you can layer in a deeper understanding of how the physical practice shifts our energetic state, too.

If storytelling is your thing, you might look at the year as a whole to map out the different festivals and celebrations. You might look at the Hindu calendar and honour events like Diwali or Navratri. But you might feel more called to honour celebrations within your own tradition, whether the tradition of your heritage or another lineage that you are connected to. The traditions local to where you are might also be the ones that students most easily relate to, and these are present for everyone in some way. For example, you can't miss that it's Valentine's Day if you're in the UK (and many other countries). As a teacher, you can choose whether you want your class to be a sanctuary – away from a celebration like this – or you might decide to bring it in but give it a yogic twist, like honouring the love story with the Self or connecting to the heart *chakra*, for example.

If you teach classes in terms rather than on a drop-in basis, this gives you a great opportunity to build on a theme, as you know all the students will be present for the whole journey you are taking together. With drop-in classes, you need to make sure each class is a fully standalone experience, even if it is within a series.

Workshops

Workshops offer a longer time to really dive deep with a theme. You have time to include many different practices within it, to speak more at length, to break down detail and to offer time for questions and discussion if you wish. At workshops, you also know that students are showing up out of their interest in the particular theme you are offering, so you can really go deep with it. In a class situation, you might have to be a bit more general, on the whole. For example, if in a class you are focusing on a particular *asana*, you may want to break down alignment points clearly; however, if your class style is *vinyasa* flow, you probably don't want to stop and workshop the points too much, as students will be expecting, to some extent, to be moving continuously. In a workshop situation, however, you will have been able to set up a clear understanding of what to expect beforehand; students will have read your detailed workshop description.

When you choose your workshop themes, you want to really find out what is of service to your students as well as what you feel passionate about sharing. People will make the extra commitment both time-wise and financially when it's something they really feel they need, but equally, the way you get people to engage is through your own enthusiasm. So I feel it's always a balance between both. You might choose to do a series of monthly workshops that tie in with each other or do workshops aligned with events through the year. I have taught New Year's Day workshops for about a decade now, and they always prove very popular. But equally, I wouldn't teach them unless I felt that it was my favourite way to start the year, too: being and practising in community. Seasonal changes are another great subject to dedicate a workshop to. And naturally, having workshop time dedicated to understanding *asana* and anatomy tends to be really popular. As a teacher, it can be incredibly rewarding to witness the breakthroughs that happen in a workshop setting when there is more time to explore, understand and absorb the material.

Retreats

At the first retreat I ever taught, I decided to explore my love for the stories about the Vedic Goddesses. I had just tried out some storytelling in my classes, which was well received, and as I was preparing for my retreat, I thought a retreat setting would be the perfect opportunity to explore this more. There are many lovely things about yoga on retreat: you have a beautiful setting, you get looked after and cooked for, you get away from all the mundane life stuff. From a teaching point of view, it is great because you have more freedom. Often you have sole access to the yoga space, which means you can be more fluid with timings; it doesn't matter if you run over a bit or want to be more spontaneous with your schedule. On the whole, you have more time, so you can get into greater detail and offer a fuller range of practices. You can really get into the rhythm of the day and offer practices that align energetically with the time of day. Another big part for me is that you have a cohesive group for a dedicated amount of time, which means that you truly are on a shared journey. So you can really build your theme and explore different aspects. At that first retreat I taught, we explored the different energies of Shakti through the different aspects of the Goddesses. Having more time meant that I could spend longer on the stories themselves and then we took them into the embodied practices. This offered so much juicy material for us to explore as a group – discussing how we related to and found affinity with the different Goddesses. Since then, I have taught many retreats over the years that have the deities and their stories as the through line; it has become one of my favourite offerings.

But, as with classes, you can theme through any of the gateways. For example, using the five elements or the *chakras* works really well with five-to-seven-day retreats, and weekends, too. It works especially well if you are in a setting that lends itself to being in direct relationship with the elements. You could take a journey through the main themes of the *Yoga Sutras* or the *Bhagavad Gita* or perhaps use the meditations in the *Vijnana Bhairava* as inspiration, or whichever scripture really speaks to your heart. Perhaps you use the *asana* as the gateway, moving through different groups of postures each day and then using the theming template to take it deeper into all aspects of the practice and contemplation.

Personally, I love retreats because of being able to dive deep. You can really feel the potency of transformation that can happen when you have dedicated time to practise. It offers the opportunity for reflection and perspective, so as a teacher, you can truly offer fertile ground for this to happen in an even more profound way. And though you might not use personal stories to theme a whole week (this would be a bit self-indulgent!), being on retreat with students offers them the opportunity to ask about your journey and personal experiences with practice. I do feel that an important part of the retreat experience is having time with fellow yoga students as well as your teacher.

— *Chapter 11*—

YOUR PERSONAL
OVERALL THEME

Your Deeper 'Why'

As teachers, what we make of our classes and what we bring to them is completely up to us. We can keep it simple or we can get as creative as we like. Ultimately, what it all comes down to is our 'why' – why are we teaching yoga? I might be wrong, but I doubt anyone ever chose to teach yoga because it seemed like a smart career choice. Most teachers go into teaching because they feel a deeper calling to share the practices that have benefitted them so immensely. The impulse to teach comes from a uniquely lived experience.

What do you feel your *dharma* as a teacher is? What is the very essence of what you want to share with your students? You might have a very clear idea of what this is already, but in case you don't, I suggest you take some time to contemplate it. Think back to what initially brought you to the practices. What got you onto the yoga mat or meditation cushion that very first time? And what was it that made you come back over and over again? It is useful to think about the things that have changed for the better since we came to yoga: what has shifted with our health, our mindset, our lives? Do you feel differently about yourself than you did before yoga? All of this will offer you clues as to your unique offering in your teaching. What moves you to teach isn't an esoteric idea but your own lived experience. There will be, if you like, a theme there, too. And just as the theme in your class becomes an anchoring point, the 'why' of your teaching is the anchoring point in a greater sense.

There is so much in the world, and in the modern, western yoga world, that can distract us and detract attention from what is truly important and of essence to our practice and teaching. We can easily become preoccupied with what other teachers are doing and what we think we should be doing. I cannot tell you how many times new teachers have come to me worried about what they should be doing on social media and concerned about not having what it takes to build a 'following'. And though social media is a very real aspect of most of our lives, we have to keep a healthy perspective. We always have a choice in how we engage. But we have to become very clear and discerning to not be consumed by overwhelm – or by the 'comparison monster'. First of all, we can fully challenge how we see yoga being portrayed on social media – are we in agreement with it? And do we want to contribute or challenge the mainstream ideas? We also want to get clear on why we engage with social media. It might be to build an audience; in which case, you need some strategy and social-media marketing acumen. However, you can also approach social media as a way to simply stay connected with your students. It's a tool for letting your community know what you are offering, and it can be an opportunity to continue to explore the themes you have been offering in your classes or workshops. In this way, you also reinforce the idea that practice continues off the mat and in life.

We can easily get distracted by what 'success' means for a yoga teacher. Does it mean packed classes? Does it mean peak time slots at a top yoga studio? Does it mean being on the cover of a yoga magazine? I think it is time to examine where these ideas come from and if they actually ring true to us. Because surely, success is completely individual? Are there any external markers of success that are really true? After all, we hear about many outwardly successful people who actually suffer greatly within. And is this not exactly where our practices can offer us support?

In the tradition, we come across the teaching of the *Purushartas*, the four paths of fulfilment in life. According to the *Purushartas*, we have four aims in life. The first is to fulfil our soul purpose or *dharma*, the second, *artha*, is the worldly support to do so. The third is pleasure and enjoyment (*kama*), and the fourth refers to spiritual liberation: *moksha*. The underlying idea is that we all come into this life with a unique purpose, and we will only find fulfilment once we align with this. This verse from the *Bhagavad Gita* feels like a good reminder to return to again and again.

> It is better to strive in one's own *dharma* than to succeed in the *dharma* of another. Nothing is ever lost following one's own *dharma*, but competition in another's *dharma* breeds fear and insecurity. *Bhagavad Gita* III.35 (Easwaran 1985, p.108)

It isn't necessarily easy to understand what our *dharma* is. We live in a culture with strong norms and expectations. We are fed ideas of what achievement and success look like from when we are young. We are also not encouraged to listen to our inner knowing. It takes a lot of practice and unravelling to do so, which in turn requires courage and commitment. In this way, I feel so strongly that yoga can be a truly revolutionary path in how it challenges dominant culture.

But finding this freedom also calls for courage. To expand ourselves beyond the expected requires tenacity. Having a sense of our purpose propels us forwards even when we meet resistance, when we push against the boundaries of the conventional. Ultimately, living our purpose is about finding where and how we are best of service to the greater whole. And this might or might not be through your career. It might be in how you offer your time to a local community garden or how you look after your family. Teaching yoga might only be part of the picture. But when you do teach yoga, it is good to have an idea of what your greater purpose with it is. This is what will help you reconnect in the moments when you feel uninspired or lost, when you're dragging yourself to class or distracted by things going on in your private life.

Here are a few journaling prompts to help you feel into your personal 'why' and *dharma* as a yoga teacher:

1. What brought me to yoga was...

2. What I found through yoga was...

3. When I practise yoga I feel…

4. My greatest wish for my students is…

Now read through what you have written and reflect on the common themes and the words that stand out as important to you. In the same way as you distilled your class themes, now distil the essence of what you have written into a short statement or even just a few words. These words need to be words that you feel resonate in your heart; this is for you, not for anyone else. It can be simple and potent.

Then, take some time to reflect on where you might serve this personal *dharma* the best. Is there a specific community that will be particularly well served by what you have to offer? Is there part of your story that will make you a great guide for a particular group of people?

I offer this here as something to feel into, as this will also be a guiding light in how you come to theme your classes. The bigger picture feeds into the smaller and vice versa.

And having a sense of purpose also helps when we falter and feel uninspired or distracted by what everyone else is offering or what we 'should' be doing. Remember, there is only one you and what you have to offer is unique and needed. Your voice and wisdom will be exactly the medicine someone out there needs. We are all offering the beautiful teachings of an ancient tradition, but the way we embody and convey it will speak differently to different people. In this way, I don't think there can ever be 'too many' yoga teachers.

Theming classes is not for everyone or for every time. There will be times when it feels really right to turn up to class with no plan and simply feel into the moment. There will be other times when less talking and simpler guidance is what is called for. The intention of this book is to offer some of the tools I have found useful in the hope that you will find them helpful, too. My greatest hope is that what I offer here has stirred some inspiration within you to reconnect to your own innate curiosity and creativity, especially, perhaps, for those moments when you might find yourself feeling a bit stuck or stale in your teaching. In my own experience, it might seem like we hit an insurmountable wall at times, but actually it doesn't need much, just a little nudge of a word of encouragement or insight and then we can feel tapped back into our creative flow.

Perhaps the most important thing to remember at any time that we feel a bit lost, confused or stuck is to go back to the source teachings. Pick up one of the scriptures or seek out one of the elders of the tradition. The ancient wisdom of this extraordinary path will guide and support you.

In honour of all the gurus, teachers, teachings and lineages of yoga ~ *Om Sri Gurubhyo Namaha.*

And now it's over to you – I hope you will enjoy filling in your theming lotus many times over!

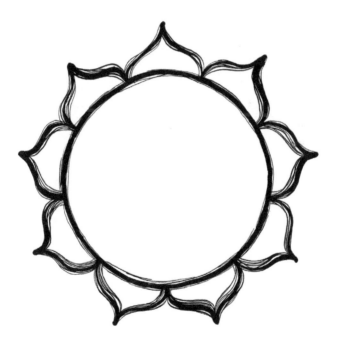

REFERENCES

Easwaran, E. (1985) *The Bhagavad Gita*. Tomales, CA: Nilgiri Press.

Easwaran, E. (1987) *The Upanishads*. Tomales, CA: Nilgiri Press.

Kempton, S. (2013) *Awakening Shakti*. Boulder, CO: Sounds True.

Stiles, M. (2002) *Yoga Sutras of Patanjali*. Boston, MA: Weiser Books.

Tigunait, P. R. (2017) *The Practice of the Yoga Sutra, Sadhana Pada*. Honesdale, PA: Himalayan Institute.

RESOURCES

Carrol, C. and Carroll, R. (2012) *Mudras of India*. London: Singing Dragon.

Desikachar, T. K. V. (1995) *The Heart of Yoga*. Rochester, VA: Inner Traditions International.

Frawley, D. (1999) *Yoga & Ayurveda*. Twin Lakes, WI: Lotus Press.

Iyengar, B. K. S. (2005) *Light on Life*. London: Rodale.

Rama, S. (1978) *Living with the Himalayan Masters*. Honesdale, PA: Himalayan Institute.

Stryker, R. (2011) *The Four Desires*. New York, NY: Random House.

Tigunait, P. R. (2002) *Inner Quest (Second Edition)*. Honesdale, PA: Himalayan Institute.

INDEX